Principles and Practice Series

RESPIRATORY MEASUREMENT

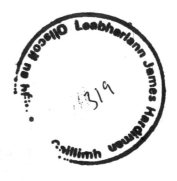

Principles and Practice Series

RESPIRATORY MEASUREMENT

GÖRAN HEDENSTIERNA
Professor of Clinical Physiology
Uppsala University, Uppsala, Sweden

Series Editors

C E W HAHN
Professor of Anaesthetic Science
University of Oxford,
and Consultant in Clinical Measurement,
Oxford Radcliffe Hospital

and

A P ADAMS
Professor of Anaesthetics,
University of London,
United Medical and Dental Schools of
Guy's and St Thomas' Hospitals
and Honorary Consultant Anaesthetist,
Guy's, King's, and St Thomas' Hospitals, London

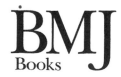

BMJ
Books

First published in 1998
by BMJ Books, BMA House, Tavistock Square,
London WC1H 9JR

British Library Cataloguing in Publication Data

A catalogue record for this book is available
from the British Library

ISBN 0-7279-1207-0

Typeset by Apek Typesetters Ltd, Nailsea, Bristol
Printed and bound in Great Britain by Latimer Trend, Plymouth

Contents

Preface

This book deals with the physiological principles of ventilation and gas exchange and the methods that can be used for assessing pulmonary function, with special emphasis on those methods that can be applied or have been modified to be applicable during anaesthesia. To this end, the first part of the book describes the function of the healthy lung, focusing on ventilation and gas exchange. Effects of chronic lung disease, both obstructive and restrictive (fibrotic), are also described.

The second part of the book is devoted to the normal as well as pathophysiological changes that may occur during anaesthesia. Special emphasis is put on the relationship between morphology and function. Acute respiratory failure, with its most severe form, acute respiratory distress syndrome, is also touched upon. This is because there are similarities between these disease states and the normal lung during anaesthesia.

Finally, the third part of the book deals with the practice of respiratory measurement, with emphasis on ventilation and volumes, mechanics of the respiratory system, and gas exchange.

It is hoped that this book can stimulate the thinking of respiratory physiology in the anaesthetised patient, and provide practical aspects on how to carry out measurements of pulmonary function during anaesthesia and muscle paralysis.

My most sincere thanks go to Birgit Andersson, who has given a huge amount of secretarial help, and to Eva-Maria Hedin who did all drawings.

Göran Hedenstierna
Uppsala, Sweden and San Diego, California

Part I

Physiological principles in health and chronic disease

The first part of this book focuses upon pulmonary physiology in the normal, healthy subject as well as in obstructive and restrictive lung disease. The physiological aspects of the lung are partitioned into the ventilation and the volumes of the lung, the mechanical characteristics of the lung and the chest wall, the distribution and diffusion of air in the airways and across the alveolar-capillary membranes, and blood flow through the pulmonary capillaries. Finally, the oxygenation of blood and elimination of carbon dioxide are discussed and causes of hypoxaemia and hypercapnia are analysed.

1: Introduction

The major task of the lung is to oxygenate the blood and eliminate carbon dioxide from it. This is accomplished by an exchange of gas between the gas in the lungs (alveolar gas) and the pulmonary capillary blood. Air is brought down into the alveoli through cyclic breathing and oxygen in the inspired gas diffuses through the alveolar epithelial wall, the interstitial tissue, and the capillary endothelial wall, as well as the plasma, finally reaching the haemoglobin inside the red blood cells. Carbon dioxide diffuses in the opposite direction, from the blood cells and the plasma to the alveolar gas phase, and is expired. To establish a gas exchange in the human lung, there must thus be ventilation of the alveoli, diffusion through the alveolar-capillary membranes, and circulation or perfusion of the pulmonary capillary bed (Fig 1.1).

Ventilation is created by movement of the rib cage and diaphragm. The upward movement of the ribs and the downward shift of the dome of the diaphragm expand the lung tissue and suck air into the alveoli. The work

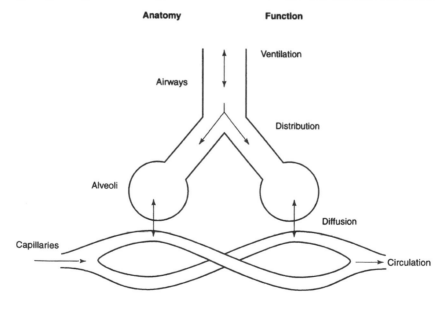

Fig 1.1   An overview of the anatomical and functional basis of the lungs.

that is required to force gas into the lungs is normally very small—1–2% of the total energy expenditure at rest.[1] Expiration is passive, that is, the elastic recoil of the lung pushes out the air without the use of the respiratory muscles. This means that the inspiratory muscles also do expiratory work, because they have to overcome the elastic recoil force of the lung during inspiration, and the energy stored in lengthened elastic fibres is released when these fibres are shortened during expiration. In lung disease and during heavy breathing, for example, during strenuous exercise, respiratory work may, however, increase dramatically and also require active effort during expiration. Respiratory work may become a limiting factor for physical exercise and even for the maintenance of basal gas exchange.[23] In the second case, ventilatory support may be needed to maintain life.

Each lung contains more than 100 million alveoli.[4] This large number requires a gas distribution system that functions well, that is, non-obstructed airways. Even with the most perfectly functioning airway system, however, gas distribution is far from even (see chapter 5). Before proceeding it is necessary to define what is meant by "even". Gas distribution is uneven in relation to the size of alveoli. More gas goes to the lower (dependent) lung areas, which have the smallest alveoli, than to upper (non-dependent) lung areas in a gravitational direction.[5] The mechanism behind this involves the difference in pleural pressure at different lung levels. This pressure is higher, less "negative", around the lower lung regions than higher up, which is an effect of the weight of the lung itself. The transpulmonary pressure, that is, the alveolar pressure (equal to atmospheric pressure at end inspiration or end expiration) minus pleural pressure, decreases down the lung as does the distension pressure of the alveoli. The more expanded an alveolus is, the greater the pressure required to expand it further. This causes the smaller, dependent alveoli to expand more during inspiration than those larger ones that are higher up.[5]

A seemingly unwanted effect of the structure of the human lung is that it causes some of the ventilation to be "wasted", that is, it will not participate in the gas exchange. This results because the part of the breath that has not reached the alveoli, but is still in the airways, may not deliver oxygen or receive carbon dioxide. This "dead space" ventilation accounts for almost a third of an ordinary tidal breath, that is, the dead space/tidal volume ratio (V_D/V_T) is close to 0·3.[6] It may be surprising that humans, whom we may think of as highly developed creatures, need to ventilate some 30% more to compensate for dead space, whereas fish do not have this re-breathing. Fish take in water through the mouth, let it flow over the gills, and then it is passed out through the gill openings, that is, the fish has a one way system. Birds have airways that are partly divided, using certain airways for inspiration and others for expiration, which reduces dead space. Why then should humans have a less sophisticated system? In fact, dead space also has important functions, besides distributing gas. It conditions inspired air by removing particles, saturating it with water vapour, and adjusting the temperature to that of the body. A lesson was learned when patients with poliomyelitis were given a chronic tracheostomy to reduce their dead space so that they could eliminate CO_2 more efficiently. Many patients developed pneumonitis as a result of the unconditioned respiratory gas, and several patients succumbed. Thus, the delicate alveolar–capillary interphase in the human lung can easily be damaged and requires conditioning of gas, accomplished by the conducting airways, or dead space. A more robust lung structure at the alveolar level could withstand unconditioned gas, but instead present a diffusion limiting barrier for respiratory gas.

Not only are the thickness and quality of the alveolar–capillary barrier of importance for gas exchange; the size of the alveolar area, available for diffusion, is also important. All alveoli together make up a surface of about 75 m^2,[4] which is not bad in view of the fact that this area is within a lung that is 3–4 litres at rest, and can be expanded to 6–8 litres. Thus, any condition that reduces alveolar surface area, for example, fibrotic disorders, atelectasis, lung resection, etc, reduces the diffusing capacity. In addition to the thickness of the membranes and the area of the alveoli, the volume of capillary blood is of importance for determining the diffusion of gas between alveoli and lung capillaries. This can easily be appreciated if it is remembered that gas will diffuse from one compartment to another as long as there is a concentration or pressure difference (gradient) between them. The larger the capillary blood volume, the greater the diffusion of gas from alveoli to capillaries. Moreover, as almost all O_2 is taken up by the haemoglobin in the red cells, a binding that no longer causes any counterpressure to diffusion, the haemoglobin concentration is an important determinant of O_2 transport across the membranes. Anaemia reduces and polycythaemia increases diffusion.[7]

Finally, blood must be pumped through the pulmonary vessels to allow a continuous diffusion of gas between the gas phase and the blood. Blood flow is not evenly distributed in the lung. Gravity causes flow to be larger in dependent, lower regions of the lung than in the upper ones.[8] This is fortunate because it causes a distribution of blood flow that is fairly similar to that of ventilation. A good match between ventilation and blood flow is necessary for optimum gas transfer, whereas even distributions in relation to the alveoli and capillary bed are less important, at least during resting conditions.[9] This may not be obvious, but what is obvious is that it is not compatible with life to ventilate one lung and perfuse the other. Atelectasis or consolidation of lung tissue by pneumonia causes blood to flow through the lung without coming into contact with ventilated lung parenchyma. This causes a shunt, or the passage through the lung of mixed venous blood that does not take up any O_2 or deliver any CO_2 to the alveoli. More common is a mismatch between ventilation and blood flow, so that some regions are better perfused than they are ventilated, for example, behind a partially obstructed airway in an asthmatic patient. These regions contribute to impaired oxygenation of the blood. Other regions may be better ventilated than perfused. They do not impair oxygenation but represent an inefficient use of ventilation and increase the ventilatory demand. These disturbances are commonly called ventilation–perfusion ($\dot{V}A/\dot{Q}$) mismatch.[9]

Another aspect of the pulmonary circulation is that it is a low pressure system. This has been achieved by the larger diameters and shorter lengths of the pulmonary vessels than of those in the systemic circulation.[4] The advantage is that the pulmonary circulation can be maintained at much lower pressures than in the systemic circulation, the systolic and diastolic pressures in the pulmonary artery being about 20 and 8 mm Hg compared with the typical 120/80 (mm Hg) in the systemic arteries. This low pressure system prevents diffusion of blood through the vessel wall, despite the thinness of the alveolar–capillary barrier. On the other hand, the system is vulnerable to a pressure increase which rapidly causes an oedema.

The lung is regularly affected by anaesthesia and mechanical ventilation in all four areas of function: ventilation, distribution, diffusion, and circulation. This already occurs in the healthy volunteer or the patient with no cardiopulmonary disease, and sometimes the dysfunction can be sufficiently severe to cause life threatening hypoxaemia. In patients with pre-existing lung disease, gas exchange will be compromised further compared with the awake state. Knowledge of the functional impairment that will ensue during anaesthesia, and during mechanical ventilation, makes ventilatory support possible which should, in the large majority of patients, prevent any disastrous impairment of gas exchange.

1 Otis AB. The work of breathing. In: Fenn WO, Rahn H, eds. *Handbook of physiology*, Section 3. *Respiration*, vol 1. Washington DC: American Physiological Society, 1964: 463–76.
2 Campbell EJM, Westlake EK, Cherniack RM. Simple methods of estimating oxygen consumption and efficiency of the muscles of breathing. *J Appl Physiol* 1957;**11**:303.
3 Milic-Emili J. Work of breathing. In: Crystal RG, West JB et al, eds. *The lung scientific foundations*, vol 1. New York: Raven Press, 1991: 1065–75.
4 Weibel ER. *Morphometry of the human lung*. Berlin: Springer Verlag, 1963.
5 Milic-Emili J. Static distribution of lung volumes. In: Macklem PT, Mead J, eds. *Handbook of physiology: mechanics of breathing*, vol 2. Bethesda, MD: American Physiologic Society, 1986: 561–74.
6 Harris EA, Hunter ME, Seelye ER, Vedder M, Whitelock RML. Prediction of the physiological dead-space in resting normal subjects. *Clin Sci* 1973;**45**:375.
7 Crapo RO, Morris AH. Standardized single breath normal values for carbon monoxide diffusing capacity. *Am Rev Respir Dis* 1981;**123**:185–9.
8 West JB, Dollery CT, Naimark A. Distribution of blood flow in isolated lung: relation to vascular and alveolar pressures. *J Appl Physiol* 1964;**19**:713–24.
9 West JB. Ventilation–perfusion relationships. *Am Rev Respir Dis* 1977;**116**:919–43.

2: Ventilation

Resting conditions

Fresh air is brought into the lungs by cyclic breathing. A normal tidal breath at rest in an adult subject is about 0·5–0·6 litre and the respiratory frequency is around 16 breaths/min, with a range from 12 to 22 breaths/min. The metabolic demand and the pulmonary function determine the precise magnitude and rate, provided that the respiratory centre in the brain stem is intact and functioning. This results in a minute ventilation of about 7–8 l/min, with a variation of 2–3 litres around the mean.

All that is inspired does not reach the alveoli. About 100–150 ml are confined to the airways and do not participate in the gas exchange. This "dead space" is thus about 30% of the tidal volume, that is, the V_D/V_T ratio is 0·3 (see Fig 2.1 for different forms of dead spaces). The remainder of ventilation reaches alveoli and respiratory bronchioles (with some alveoli tapered on the airway wall). Thus, the "alveolar ventilation" is around

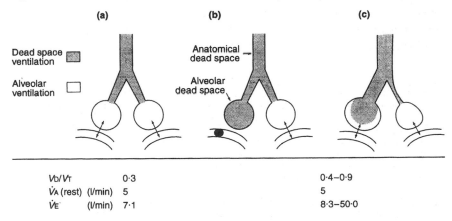

		(a)	(c)
V_D/V_T		0·3	0·4–0·9
$\dot{V}_A$ (rest)	(l/min)	5	5
$\dot{V}_E$	(l/min)	7·1	8·3–50·0

Fig 2.1 Dead space and alveolar ventilation in (a) normal and (b, c) diseased lungs: (b) pulmonary embolus; (c) chronic obstructive pulmonary disease. Note that both cessation of blood flow and excessive alveolar ventilation relative to perfusion cause an increase in dead space, as measured with a conventional CO_2 elimination technique. See also the marked increase in minute ventilation that is required to maintain alveolar ventilation when dead space is increased. V_D/V_T, ratio of dead space : tidal volume $\dot{V}_A$, alveolar ventilation; $\dot{V}_E$, minute ventilation (sum of dead space and alveolar ventilations).

5 l/min, similar to the cardiac output which is also some 5 l/min. The overall alveolar ventilation–perfusion ratio is thus 1.

There are several causes of an increased minute ventilation, such as physical exercise, reduced inspired oxygen concentration (or, rather, partial pressure of O_2), increased dead space ventilation, and metabolic acidosis.

Hyperventilation and exercise

It is possible voluntarily to increase minute ventilation to a maximum that is almost twentyfold higher than resting ventilation, to over 100 l/min in women and over 150 l/min in men, but only for a brief period of half a minute or so.[1] In addition, hyperventilation without a simultaneous increase in metabolic demand lowers the arterial partial pressure of CO_2 ($Pa\text{co}_2$) and affects consciousness. In respiratory tests of ventilatory capacity, it is therefore necessary to do the test during re-breathing of expired gas, or add CO_2 to the respiratory gas, so as to maintain the $Pa\text{co}_2$ at a normal or near normal level. The increase in ventilation is brought about by an increase in the tidal volume, to about two thirds of the vital capacity (see below), or 2·5–4 litres, and an increase in the frequency to 40 breaths/min or more. During maximum physical exercise, however, minute ventilation increases less, to around two thirds of the maximum capacity. This means an increase to 65–100 l/min in normally fit women and men. In athletes the ventilation may exceed 150 l/min.

Ventilation increases more than cardiac output during exercise

It is interesting to note that the increase in ventilation ($\dot{V}$) during exercise is far larger than the simultaneous increase in cardiac output. The increase in cardiac output is typically 5 l/min at rest, and increases to a maximum of around 25 l/min in a normally fit person (Table 2.1),[2] that is, "only" a

Table 2.1 Ventilatory and circulatory variables at rest and during maximum exercise in normally fit, healthy subjects

	Rest	Exercise*
$\dot{V}_E$ (l/min)	7	100 (150)
V_T (l)	0·5	2·5 (3·7)
f (l/min)	14	40
CO (l/min)	5	25
SV (ml)	70	150
HR (/min)	70	170

$\dot{V}_E$, minute ventilation; V_T, tidal volume; f, respiratory frequency; CO, cardiac output; SV, stroke volume; HR, heart rate.
Numbers within parentheses show maximal voluntary ventilation and tidal volume during a short test period (15–30 s).

fivefold increase! The larger increase in ventilation cannot be explained by the dead space ventilation, which "steals" from the air going down to the alveoli for gas exchange. Dead space also increases with the increase in ventilation, but hardly in proportion to the increase in tidal volume, so that the dead space to tidal volume ratio, if anything, is reduced from its resting value of around 0·3 to 0·2 or less. There is another difference between the ventilation and circulation, however, and that is the extraction of O_2 from the alveolar gas and systemic blood. During air breathing, the inspired O_2 concentration is almost 21%, and at rest the expired concentration is typically 17%. During maximum exercise, the expired O_2 concentration is reduced to around 12–13%. In other words, the extraction of O_2 has increased from 4% to 8–9% of the inspired air, or the minute ventilation. The extraction of O_2 from the blood is greater than from the air at rest, and this difference increases further during exercise. Thus, the saturation of systemic arterial blood is normally 98%, and that of mixed venous blood 75%. During heavy exercise, arterial saturation remains high whereas venous saturation is further reduced, to 10–15% in the extreme case.[2] Thus, the extraction has increased from 23% at rest to 83–88% during maximum physical effort, that is, more than 3·5 times.

Ventilation of hypoxic gas

If there is less O_2 in the inspired air, for example, living at a high altitude, alveolar and arterial Po_2 are reduced. How alveolar Po_2 can be calculated is shown in Table 2.2. At an altitude of 2400 m (8000 feet), corresponding to that of Mexico City, Pio_2 (inspired oxygen tension) is 14·4 kPa (108 mm Hg) and, at a normal $Paco_2$ of 5·32 kPa (40 mm Hg), the Pao_2 can be calculated as 7·7 kPa (58 mm Hg). By hyperventilation, $Paco_2$ can be reduced to, say, 4 kPa (30 mm Hg), with a resulting Pao_2 of 9·3 kPa (70 mm Hg). This may be sufficient to maintain a Pao_2 above 8·7 kPa (65 mm Hg), because there is also an alveolar–arterial gradient of a few millimetres of mercury. How much more is it necessary to ventilate to lower $Paco_2$ down to 4 kPa (30 mm Hg)? This can be calculated using the alveolar gas equation shown in the box on page 142. Here it may suffice to say that there is a reciprocal relationship between $Paco_2$ and V_A; $Paco_2$ will be changed to the same extent as, but in the opposite direction to, the change in V_A. Thus, to create a change in $Paco_2$ from 5·3 to 4 kPa (40 to 30 mm Hg), V_A has to increase from 30 to 40 ventilation units, or by 33%. Assuming a constant V_D/V_T, minute ventilation has to be increased to the same extent.

The situation is worse for anyone who climbs Mount Everest to the top (8848 m) and insists on breathing atmospheric air. The atmospheric pressure was measured with a barometer brought up to the summit during an expedition in 1981.[3] Barometric pressure (Pb) was indeed higher than

9

anticipated: 253 mm Hg (33·7 kPa) compared with 236 mm Hg, possibly an effect of the huge land mass of the Himalayas. Still, the corresponding P_{IO_2} was no higher than 5·8 kPa (43·3 mm Hg), which results in a negative (or zero) P_{AO_2} during quiet breathing (P_{aCO_2} of 5·3 kPa or 40 mm Hg). Ventilation will, however, be excessive at the top, and an expired air sample, collected on the summit of Mount Everest during the expedition of 1981, showed an end tidal P_{CO_2} of as low as 1 kPa (7·5 mm Hg)! This results in a P_{AO_2} of 4·7 kPa (35 mm Hg). At this low pressure, diffusion of oxygen across the alveolar–capillary membranes will be impeded, to make things worse. The calculated P_{aO_2} at the summit of Mount Everest was as low as 3·7 kPa (28 mm Hg). The ventilation needed to lower P_{aCO_2} down to 1 kPa (7·5 mm Hg) was not measured on the top of Mount Everest. By using the alveolar gas equation, however, the alveolar ventilation must be increased almost six times to lower P_{aCO_2} from 5·3 to 0·93 kPa (40 to 7 mm Hg) at a basal CO_2 elimination. As considerable effort is expended to reach the summit, the O_2 demand or consumption ($\dot{V}_{O_2}$) and CO_2 excretion or

Table 2.2   Barometric pressure relative to altitude

Altitude (metres)	Barometric pressure		Inspired P_{O_2}	
	(kPa)	(mm Hg)	(kPa)	(mm Hg)
0	101·3	760	19·9	149
250	98·4	738	19·3	144
500	95·5	716	18·7	140
750	92·6	695	18·1	135
1 000	89·9	674	17·4	131
1 500	84·6	635	16·3	123
2 000	79·5	596	15·3	115
2 500	74·7	560	14·3	107
3 000	70·1	526	13·4	101
3 500	65·8	494	12·4	93
4 000	61·6	462	11·5	87
4 500	57·7	433	10·7	80
5 000	54·0	405	9·9	75
5 500	50·6	380	9·2	69
6 000	47·2	354	8·5	64
6 500	44·2	331	7·9	59
7 000	41·1	308	7·3	55
7 500	38·4	288	6·7	51
8 000	35·6	267	6·2	46
8 500	33·2	249	5·6	42
9 000	30·7	230	5·1	38
9 500	28·6	214	4·6	35
10 000	26·4	198	4·2	32
12 000	19·3	145	2·8	21
14 000	14·1	106	1·7	12
16 000	10·3	77	0·9	7
18 000	7·5	56	0·3	2
20 000	5·5	41	0·0	0

From *Manual of ICAO Standard Atmosphere.*[6]

production ($\dot{V}_{CO_2}$) must have been increased. In theoretical calculations, the O_2 uptake was assumed to be 350 ml/min—a very modest increase compared with a basal uptake of about 250 ml/min.[3] Thus, ventilation may have been increased to at least 50 l/min (basal metabolic rate) and more probably to 75–100 l/min, taking into account the physical exercise ($1·4 \times$ basal metabolic rate [assuming $\dot{V}_{CO_2}$ to increase as much as $\dot{V}_{O_2}$], $\times 6$, to lower P_{aCO_2} to 1 kPa or 7·5 mm Hg). The reason for assuming only a modest increase in $\dot{V}_{O_2}$ is simply because P_{aO_2} and mixed venous P_{CO_2} would drop to values that are hardly compatible with life if $\dot{V}_{O_2}$ were to increase further.

Increased dead space ventilation

If dead space is increased, ventilation must be raised to account for the "losses" and to maintain P_{aCO_2} at a normal level. Dead space is increased when ventilation is through a mouthpiece and a valve or through a facemask. This "apparatus dead space" is between 25 ml and a few hundred millilitres, compared with the 100–150 ml that the natural airways make up ("anatomical dead space").[4] Bronchiectasis increases the anatomical dead space, but it adds very little to the total figure. A much larger increase can be caused by ventilation of alveoli that are not perfused, for example, a pulmonary embolus stopping blood flow of a lung unit ("alveolar dead space") (see Fig 2.1). A worst case is a plugging of the right or left main pulmonary artery, leaving one lung essentially non-perfused. In this case the dead space fraction is doubled from the normal 0·3 to 0·6 or so.[5] Patients with recurrent emboli, or pulmonary embolism, often have high V_D/V_T ratios, which can exceed 0·7–0·8. This means that, to maintain an ordinary alveolar ventilation of 5 l/min, minute ventilation must be raised from 7–8 to 20 l/min. Patients with recurrent emboli also frequently complain of dyspnoea, even in the absence of any severe hypoxaemia— because of the increased ventilatory demand. Other patients who have increased dead space are those with obstructive lung disease, for example, asthma, chronic bronchitis, and emphysema. Their major difficulty is that some regions are poorly ventilated as a result of airway obstruction, so that these regions are underventilated in relation to their perfusion, commonly called a ventilation–perfusion mismatch ("$\dot{V}_A/\dot{Q}$" mismatch signified by low $\dot{V}_A/\dot{Q}$ ratios). This forces inspired air to other regions which may be ventilated in excess of their perfusion. Such opposite $\dot{V}_A/\dot{Q}$ mismatch (signified by high $\dot{V}_A/\dot{Q}$ ratios) has the same effect on alveolar ventilation and gas exchange as an increase in dead space, and is also measured as a dead space, using standard techniques (dealt with later) (see Fig. 2.1). Indeed, a patient with advanced chronic bronchitis may have a V_D/V_T ratio as high as 0·8–0·9. Such patients would have to ventilate some 30–50 l/min to maintain a normal P_{aCO_2}, a difficult task to perform even for a short period with healthy lungs. It should therefore come as no surprise that Pa_{CO_2} goes up as a measure of alveolar "hypoventilation". This has led to the belief, erroneously, that bronchitic patients are hypoventilating when in fact they may be hyperventilating! According to the alveolar gas equation (see Table 18.1), CO_2 can be excreted by half the "normal" alveolar ventilation if Pa_{CO_2} is doubled.

As all subjects, even those with the most healthy lungs, do have some $\dot{V}_A/\dot{Q}$ mismatch, the sum of anatomical and alveolar dead spaces, whether the result of emboli or uneven ventilation and perfusion, is called "physiological dead space".

1 Quanjer PH, Tammeling GJ. Standardized lung function testing. *Bull Eur Physiopathol Respir* 1983;**19**(suppl 5):7–10.
2 Bevegård BS, Sheperd JT. Regulation of the circulation during exercise in man. *Physiol Rev* 1967;**47**:178–213.
3 West JB, Hackett PH, Maret KH, Milledge JS, Peters RM, Pizzo CJ, Winslow RM. Pulmonary gas exchange on the summit of Mount Everest. *J Appl Physiol: Respir Environ Exercise Physiol* 1983;**55**:678–87.
4 Fowler WS. Lung function studies. IV. Postural changes in respiratory dead space and functional residual capacity. *J Clin Invest* 1950;**29**:1437.
5 Severinghaus JW, Stupfel M. Alveolar dead space as an index of distribution of blood flow in pulmonary capillaries. *J Appl Physiol* 1957;**10**:335.
6 ICAO. *Manual of ICAO Standard Atmosphere*. International Civil Aviation Organization (ICAO), Montréal, Canada 1964. Doc. 788/2.

3: Lung volumes

Functional residual capacity

There is a certain amount of air in the lungs after an ordinary expiration. This volume is called the functional residual capacity (FRC). It amounts to about 3–4 litres, and is dependent on sex, age, height, and weight. It goes up with height and down with age and weight, and is smaller in women than in men.[1] The volume is determined by the balance of the inwardly directed forces of the lung ("elastic recoil", which actually consists not only of the elastic fibres of the lung tissue, but also the contractile forces of airway smooth muscles and the surface tension of alveoli), and the outwardly directed forces exerted by the ribs, joints, and muscles which make up the chest wall. It can be asked why there is a persisting gas volume in the lung after an expiration. There are at least two good reasons: one is that, if alveoli collapse during expiration, much more effort would have to be spent on re-opening them again than during a normal breath with no collapse. This is because the liquid–gas interphase in an open lung unit causes less resistance when expanding an alveolar wall than breaking a liquid–liquid interphase. The other reason is that the inspired air mixes with the remaining gas in the lung, levelling off the variation in O_2 and CO_2 concentrations that occurs during the respiratory cycle. With only a small amount of air in the lung, the gas variations in the alveoli would be much greater and would cause a similarly varying Pao_2 and $Paco_2$ in the blood. This can indeed be seen in patients with reduced FRC (see below for examples).

With increased ventilation, as during exercise, tidal volume is increased by increasing both inspiration and expiration so that the FRC is lowered by about 0·5 litre. In the presence of airway obstruction, however, as, for example, in asthma, expiration is slowed down so that the end expiratory level is elevated instead of lowered.[2] This is called air trapping and is a means of reducing the resistance to airflow in the narrowed airways. It has to be paid for because the increased breathing level increases the elastic work of breathing (see chapter 9).

In chronic obstructive lung disease, over the years the FRC increases faster than in normal people.[3] This may be an effect of chronic air trapping and loss of elastic lung tissue, which lessens the contractile forces of the lung and moves the balancing point between the outward forces of the chest wall and the inward forces of the lung to a new, higher lung volume (Fig 3.1).

In lung disease with fibrosis of the lung, such as idiopathic fibrosis, and pneumoconiosis, as well as different forms of granulomatosis and vasculitis,

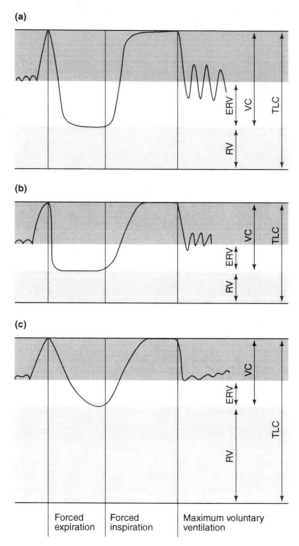

Fig 3.1 Ventilation and lung volumes in (a) a healthy subject with normal lungs, (b) a patient with restrictive lung disease (fibrosis), and (c) a patient with emphysema. Note the decrease in vital capacity (VC) and the increased expiratory flow (steeper than normal slope of the forced expiratory curve) in the fibrotic patient (b). Note also the increased residual volume (RV) and reduction in VC, and the slow forced expiration in the obstructive, emphysematous patient (c). This patient demonstrates air trapping during hyperventilation.

14

the FRC is reduced.[4] In extreme cases, the reduction can be down to 1·5–2 litres (Fig 3.1). Obviously, pulmonectomy, for example, as a treatment of lung cancer will also reduce the FRC. The remaining lung will, however, expand and fill in some of the space left after the resection of lung tissue, sometimes called "compensatory emphysema".

Total lung capacity and subdivisions

The gas volume in the lung after a maximum inspiration is called the total lung capacity (TLC). Typically, it is 6–8 litres. It can be increased in chronic obstructive lung disease, either by overexpansion or "hyper-inflation" of essentially normal alveoli, or by destruction of the alveolar wall with loss of elastic tissue, as in emphysema.[3] In extreme cases, the TLC can be increased by 50%, or to 11–12 litres. In restrictive disorders, the TLC is reduced in proportion to the severity of the fibrotic process (Fig 3.1).[4]

Even after a maximum expiratory effort, some air is left in the lung and no region normally collapses. This persisting gas volume is called residual volume (RV) and amounts to 2–2·5 litres. The reason why expiration stops before all gas has been evacuated seems to be twofold: first, distal airways sized 2 mm or less close before alveoli collapse.[5] This trapping of gas thus prevents the alveoli from being squeezed to emptiness. Second, the chest wall, rib cage, and diaphragm cannot be distorted to the point that all gas in the lung has been expelled. The advantage of not allowing lung tissue to collapse has been dealt with above (Fig 3.1).

The maximum volume that can be inspired and expired is called the vital capacity (VC). It is thus the difference between the TLC and the RV and is about 4–6 litres. It is reduced in restrictive lung diseases, frequently before a decrease in the RV. What may not be equally clear is that the VC is also reduced in obstructive lung disease. This is an effect of the chronic "air trapping" which increases the RV, mainly at the expense of the VC.[3] As mentioned above, however, the TLC may also increase, but not in proportion to the rise in the RV. The net effect can be a TLC of 12 litres, made up of an RV of 11 litres and a VC as small as 1 litre, in an extreme example of emphysema.

1 Quanjer PH, Tammeling GJ. Standardized lung function testing. *Bull Eur Physiopathol Respir* 1983;**19**(suppl 5):7–10.
2 McFadden ER Jr. Asthma: airway dynamics, cardiac function and clinical correlates. In: Middleton E Jr, Reed CE, Ellis EF, eds. *Allergy principles and practice*, 2nd edn. St Louis: CV Mosby, 1983: 843–62.
3 Pride NB, Macklem PT. Lung mechanics in disease. In: Fishman AP, Macklem PT, Mead J, Greiger SR, eds. *Handbook of physiology*. Section 3, *The respiratory system*, vol III. Bethesda, MD: American Physiological Society, 1986: 659–92.
4 Schlueter DP, Inmekus J, Stead WW. Relationship between maximal inspiratory pressure

and total lung capacity (coefficient of retraction) in normal subjects and in patients with emphysema, asthma and diffuse pulmonary infiltration. *Am Rev Respir Dis* 1967;**96**:656–65.

5 Leith DE, Mead J. Mechanisms determining residual volume of the lungs in normal subjects. *J Appl Physiol* 1967;**23**:221–7.

4: Compliance, resistance, and inductance

General

Understanding the mechanics of the respiratory system serves at least two purposes: (1) it gives the clue to what governs the distribution of inspired air, and (2) the recording of the mechanics can be used as a diagnostic and prognostic tool in lung disease. In this chapter, a start is made with an analysis of the elastic and resistive forces that have to be overcome during breathing and how these are affected by pulmonary disorders. Then the influence of the respiratory mechanics on the distribution of inspired air is analysed.

Compliance of the respiratory system

The lung recoils as an elastic rubber balloon, so a certain pressure is required to keep it inflated. The pressure needed to keep the lung inflated at a certain volume is the pleural pressure minus the alveolar pressure, or the "transpulmonary pressure" (Ptp). It will be seen that more and more pressure is required for a given volume increment the more the lung is inflated[1] (Fig 4.1). Such a curved pressure–volume relationship is typical for elastic structures, and a similar curved force–length relationship is also seen for a rubber-band.

The elastic behaviour of the lung is often analysed in terms of compliance which is the inverse of elastance. Thus, compliance (c) is expressed as a change in lung volume (ΔV), divided by the change in pressure (ΔP) that is required to cause the volume increment (or the decrease in pressure that is accompanying a volume decrement):

$$C = \Delta V / \Delta P$$

A normal lung compliance is about 0·2–0·3 l/cm H_2O (2–3 l/kPa).[1] It varies with lung volume, as can be seen from Fig 4.1, and decreases with an increase in lung volume. Thus, the compliance will be critically dependent on the lung volume at which it is measured. This should be remembered if repeated recordings are made to follow the progress of a disease. Also, if a lung, or part of it, is resected, the measured compliance is reduced despite

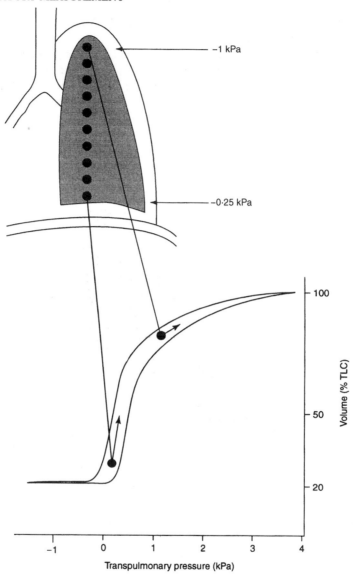

Fig 4.1 The pressure–volume relationships of the lung. Note the curved relationship which is typical for an elastic structure. Note also the lower (more subatmospheric) pleural pressure in the upper regions. The regional trans-pulmonary pressure (mouth pressure minus pleural pressure) is thus higher for apical lung units than for basal ones in an upright subject. This results in different positions of upper and lower lung regions on the pressure–volume curve. The consequence is that lower lung regions expand more for a given increase in transpulmonary pressure than upper regions. Thus, ventilation goes preferably to lower lung regions.

18

the fact that the remaining lung tissue is unaltered. This will be discussed in more detail in chapter 16.

In fibrotic lung disease, compliance is reduced and the pressure–volume curve is flatter and shifted to the right, as shown in Fig 4.2. (Obviously, the direction of a change of the pressure–volume curve depends on which axis denotes pressure and which volume; Fig 4.2 shows the standard drawing.[1]) Although the curve is sensitive to changes in the elastic properties of the lung, it is not good at discriminating between different diseases. Thus, idiopathic fibrosis, alveolar proteinosis, a granulomatosis like sarcoidosis, and interstitial and alveolar oedema all lower compliance and cause a

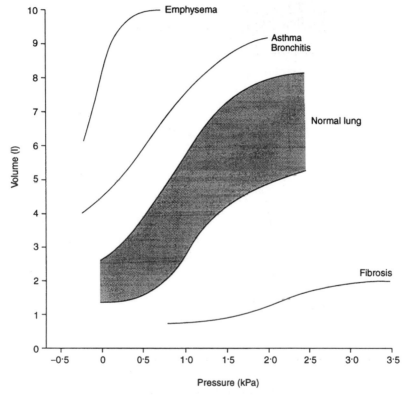

Fig 4.2 Examples of pressure–volume curves of the lung in health and in lung disease. Note the much flatter slope of the curve in fibrotic lung disease which causes considerable increase in the pressure variation and the respiratory work. Also, note the parallel shift of the pressure–volume curve of an asthmatic and bronchitic patient, showing that the compliance need not change in these diseases, although lung volume may have increased. Finally, note the steep slope of the curve of an emphysematous patient. This indicates loss of elastic tissue and might even suggest reduced respiratory work. Such patients, and asthmatic and bronchitic patients as well, have, however, an increased airway resistance which causes elevation of respiratory work.

19

flattening and right shift of the pressure–volume curve.

Loss of elastic lung tissue, as in emphysema, causes a steeper curve, which is shifted to the left[1] (Fig 4.2). Similar changes are not seen in chronic bronchitis or asthma. Thus, the recording of the pressure–volume curve can help in establishing the diagnosis of emphysema which cannot easily be done on a conventional chest radiograph. The over-aeration that can be seen on the radiograph does not enable a distinction to be made between obstructive lung disease with and that without loss of elastic tissue. With high resolution computed tomography, however, a new tool has become available for differential diagnosis.[2]

The chest wall itself also exerts an elastic impedance on breathing, which goes undetected during spontaneous breathing, because the chest wall is part of the pump itself. Chest wall mechanics can be measured in trained volunteers, but it requires tricky respiratory manoeuvres with complete relaxation of the respiratory muscles.[1] During artificial ventilation and muscle relaxation, on the other hand, the compliance of the chest wall can be measured. This is because the respiratory muscles are allowed to rest so that the rib cage and diaphragm exert elastic impedance only when the lungs are inflated and the chest wall expanded. The change in lung volume, divided by the change in pleural pressure, then gives the chest wall compliance:

$$Ccw = \Delta V/\Delta Ppl.$$

It can be seen that the compliance of the chest wall is of about the same magnitude as that of the lungs—about 0.2 l/cm H_2O (2 l/kPa). It may go down in obesity and in conditions with general oedema, as well as in disorders affecting the joints, for example, ankylosing spondylitis.[1]

Resistance of the respiratory system

Pressure is required to overcome the resistance to airflow through the airways during respiration. In addition, the sliding of different components of the lung tissue, and of the chest wall, during inspiration and expiration also exert reistance.[3] The resistance is calculated as the driving pressure divided by airflow. Flow can be measured at the airway opening, the mouth, or the nose, and is assumed to apply to all three resistances (in the airways, lung tissue, and chest wall). The driving pressure differs for resistances of the airway, lung tissue, and chest wall. The one for airway resistance is mouth (or nose) pressure minus alveolar pressure, whereas the other driving pressures will be part of the transpulmonary and pleural pressure changes, as discussed in chapter 17.

Airflow can be either turbulent, with a disorderly pattern signified by vortices, or laminar, with a streamlined unidirectional flow pattern, as seen

20

in a cross directional view. Turbulent flow is proportional to the square of the pressure, and laminar flow, which is less pressure demanding, is linearly related to the pressure. Flow is turbulent in larger airways and at bifurcations and irregularities of the bronchi, and laminar in the smaller airways. Thus, most of the energy, or pressure, needed to create an airflow is required to overcome the resistance in the larger airways.[4] In the normal subject, only about 20% of the measured airway resistance is located in the small bronchi. A doubling of "peripheral" or "small" airway resistance may indeed be difficult to detect by standard recording techniques. The difficulty in detecting changes in small airways that are roughly 2 mm wide, and less, has coined the expression "the lung's silent zone".

Airflow resistance is normally around 1 cm H_2O/l per s. It is increased in obstructive lung disease to around 5 cm H_2O/l per s in mild to moderate asthma and bronchitis, and above 10 in more severe cases.[5] It is worth noticing that breathing through an endotracheal tube size 8 causes a resistance of 5 cm H_2O/l per s at a flow of 1 l/s, and a tube of size 7 increases the resistance to 8 cm H_2O/l per s, that is, comparable to moderate asthma![6]

Airflow resistance can be higher during expiration than during inspiration, in particular during forced breathing and in patients with obstructive lung disease. This is because the expiratory muscle effort acts not only on alveoli, to empty them, but also on airways, making them narrower.[3] The inspiratory effort, on the other hand, helps to dilate airways within the thorax, by lowering the pleural pressure which acts on the outside of the airway wall. Finally, those airways that are not in the thoracic cavity, that is, pharynx, larynx, and trachea, are subject to a lower pressure inside than outside their wall during inspiration, because they are surrounded by atmospheric pressure whereas the luminal pressure is below atmospheric (otherwise no air would be sucked into that point of the airway tree).[3] These physiological consequences can also be used to separate an increase in extrathoracic resistance from an increase in resistance of other airways. If resistance is increased during inspiration, it is probably caused by narrowing of extrathoracic airways, for example, the sucking into the centre of the lumen of a paralytic vocal fold. Intraction (caused by sucking in as a result of a lower subatmospheric pressure inside the wall) of upper airways can also be seen in a neonate with respiratory distress, causing strenuous breathing.

The resistance of the lung tissue and the chest wall has been studied much less. The lung tissue resistance amounts to about 1 cm H_2O/l per s in the normal case and can be increased three- to fourfold in chronic lung disease.[7] Even less has been done about study of the chest wall resistance. It does seem, however, as though the sum of lung tissue and chest wall resistance is increased, and markedly so, in acute respiratory failure demanding mechanical ventilation.[8]

Inertance or acceleration of gas and tissue

There is finally one more component of the total impedance to breathing, and that is the inductance, or pressure required to accelerate air and tissue during inspiration and expiration. This part is, however, minor and can hardly be measured under normal breathing, whether the lungs are healthy or not. During very rapid breathing, such as high frequency oscillation in intensive care, or the yogi exercise of rapid shallow breathing of around 4 breaths/second, acceleration becomes more important and can contribute 5–10% of the total impedance to breathing.[9]

1 Agostoni E, Hyatt RE. Static behavior of the respiratory system. In: *Handbook of physiology.* Section 3, *The respiratory system*, Vol III. Bethesda, MD: American Physiological Society, 1986: 113–30.
2 Hruban RH, Meziane MA, Zerhouni EA, et al. High resolution computed tomography of inflation fixed lungs: pathologic–radiologic correlation of centrilobular emphysema. *Am Rev Respir Dis* 1987;**136**:935–40.
3 Ingram RH, Pedley TJ. Pressure–flow relationships in the lungs. In: Macklem PT, Mead J, eds. *Handbook of physiology*, Section 3: *The respiratory system*, vol III. *Mechanics of breathing.* Baltimore, MA: Williams & Wilkins, 1986: 277–93.
4 Despas P, LeRoux M, Macklem PT. Site of airway obstruction in asthma as determined by measuring maximal expiratory flow breathing air and helium–oxygen mixture. *J Clin Invest* 1972;**51**:3235–43.
5 McFadden ER Jr. Asthma: airway dynamics, cardiac function and clinical correlates. In: Middleton E Jr, Reed CE, Ellis EF, eds. *Allergy principles and practice*, 2nd edn. St Louis: CV Mosby, 1983: 843–62.
6 Holst M, Striem J, Hedenstierna G. Errors in tracheal pressure recording in patients with a tracheostomy tube: a model study. *Intensive Care Med* 1990;**16**:384–9.
7 Verbeken EK, Cauberghs M, Mertens I, Lauweryns JM, Van de Woestijne KP. Tissue and airway impedance of excised normal, senile and emphysematous lungs. *J Appl Physiol* 1992;**72**:2343–53.
8 Tantucci C, Corbeil C, Chasse M, Braidy J, Matar N, Milic-Emili J. Flow resistance in patients with chronic obstructive pulmonary disease in acute respiratory failure. Effects of flow and volume. *Am Rev Respir Dis* 1991;**144**:384–9.
9 Frostell C, Pande J, Hedenstierna G. Effects of high frequency breathing on pulmonary ventilation and gas exchange. *J Appl Physiol* 1983;**55**:1374–8.

5: Gas distribution

Distribution of inspired gas: effect of compliance, resistance, and airway closure

The air that is inspired is not evenly distributed in the lung. During quiet breathing, most goes to the lower, dependent regions, that is, basal, diaphragmatic areas in the upright or sitting position, and to dorsal units in the supine position.[1] This also means that the lower, left lung will receive most of the air if the subject is in the left lateral position, and the right lung is preferentially ventilated in the right position. The reason for this seemingly gravitational orientation of something as light as air is the combined effect of the curved pressure–volume relationship of the lung tissue and the increasing pleural pressure down the lung. This is discussed in this chapter at some length.

First, the curved pressure–volume curve, typical for an elastic tissue, means that, with increasing lung volume, more and more pressure is required to inflate the lung by a given volume increment. Second, the increasing pleural pressure, at constant alveolar pressure throughout the lungs, causes transpulmonary pressure to decrease from the top to the bottom of the lung. In the upright position, apical lung regions are exposed to a higher transpulmonary pressure than dependent, basal ones. Thus, the upper and lower lung regions are positioned at different levels of the pressure–volume curve (see Fig 4.1). During inspiration, pleural pressure is lowered, causing lower lung regions to inflate more than the upper ones, for a similar change in transpulmonary pressure (assuming that pleural pressure changes uniformly in the pleural space).[1] Thus, in healthy subjects, ventilation is preferentially to the basal regions (Fig 5.1).

The pleural pressure gradient is oriented in a vertical, gravitational direction, which is why ventilation distribution changes with body position. What causes the pleural pressure gradient? The major factor is the weight of the lung itself, with less lung tissue exerting a pressure at a level higher up in the thoracic cavity than at a lower lung level. This pressure is mediated in all directions, and also to the pleural space. The specific density of an air filled and perfused lung is, on average, about 0·3, and this causes the pleural pressure to increase by 0·3 cm H_2O/cm vertical distance. If the lung is heavier, as when there is oedema, the pleural pressure gradient increases, as does the vertical difference in alveolar size. If weight is reduced or eliminated, as at zero gravity or microgravity, there should be no vertical pleural pressure gradient, and lung expansion as well as gas distribution should be more even. This was studied during flights made in the NASA Space Laboratory and, indeed, showed a more homogeneous ventilation.[2] Some inhomogeneity persisted, however, indicating that non-gravitational factors also contribute to the ventilation distribution. These may be uneven convectional and diffusional flows in small lung units.[3]

It also seems that the vertical pleural pressure gradient is smaller in the prone position, compared with supine.[4] This possibly results from the weight of the heart which is compressing the dependent parts of the lung in the supine position, permitting the non-dependent regions to expand. In the prone position, the heart is resting on the sternum with no or minor effects on the shape of the lung. The only force that can distort the shape of the lung is the weight of the lung itself. This may result in more even distribution of inspired gas in the prone position.

So far, we have dealt with a distribution of inspired gas during, from a technical and puristic point of view, static conditions (which, however, would not result in any airflow). The distribution is essentially the same during quiet breathing, up to a flow rate of 0·5 l/s or so. With increasing flow rate, however, regional differences in airway resistance (and in lung tissue and possibly to some extent chest wall resistance—disregarded here)

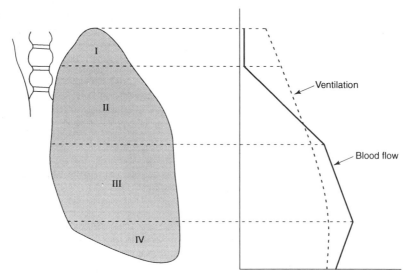

Fig 5.1   The vertical distributions of ventilation and blood flow in the lung. The so called zones I, II, III, and IV are indicated (for further details, see the text). Note that both ventilation and blood flow increase down the lung but that there is more ventilation than perfusion in the upper regions (causing a dead space like effect, or "high" $\dot{V}_A/\dot{Q}$ regions), and that perfusion exceeds ventilation in the lower lung regions, causing slight impairment of oxygenation of blood (venous admixture or "low" $\dot{V}_A/\dot{Q}$ regions).

play an increasing role in determining the gas distribution. As the lung tissue, both alveoli and airways, is more expanded in upper regions than in lower, resistance to airflow is less in the upper part of the lung. This results in a change in the distribution pattern with more gas going to upper units.[5] At a flow of 0·3 l/s, two thirds of ventilation went to the lower half of the lung, as assessed using an isotope technique, and, when inspiratory flow was increased to 4–5 l/s, distribution between the upper and lower half of the lung was even (Fig 5.2). This is advantageous for optimising the gas transfer in the lung, as, for example, during exercise, because the alveolar–capillary surface area will be more efficiently used. This postulates that perfusion distribution is evenly distributed. Perfusion does indeed adjust in the same way as ventilation, and is discussed later in this chapter.

Airways become narrower during expiration, as can be inferred from the discussion above. If expiration is deep enough, airways in dependent regions will eventually close. The volume above the residual volume (RV) at which airways begin to close during an expiration is called the closing volume (CV), and the sum of the RV and the CV is called the closing capacity (CC).[6] Airway closure is a normal physiological phenomenon and is the effect of an increasing pleural pressure during expiration. When pleural pressure becomes "positive" (or, rather, above atmospheric), it exceeds the pressure inside the airway which is almost atmospheric at low flow rates. The higher pressure outside than inside compresses the airway and closes it. As pleural pressure is higher in dependent regions than higher up, closure of the airways starts at the bottom of the lung. The crucial point is therefore the creation of a "positive" pleural pressure. In young people it may not occur until they have expired to RV. With increasing age, however, pleural pressure becomes "positive" at higher and higher lung volumes, and at an age of 65–70 years airway closure may occur above the functional residual capacity (FRC).[6] This means that, in elderly patients, dependent lung regions are intermittently closed during the breath. These regions will re-open during inspiration, when the lung volume exceeds the closing capacity. The impediment of ventilation caused by the closure of airways seems to be the main explanation for decreasing arterial oxygenation with age.

Airway closure plays an even greater role in the supine position. This is because the FRC is reduced, whereas the CC is not affected by body position. Closure of airways may occur above the FRC, at an age of 45–50 and, in the 70 year old patient, airways may be continuously closed if the CC exceeds the FRC plus the tidal volume. This is illustrated in Fig 5.3.

Airway closure occurs at higher lung volumes in patients with obstructive lung disease. Secretions, oedema of the airway wall, and increased bronchial muscle tone all reduce the lumen of the airway, facilitating premature closure of the airway.[7] As these changes are considered to start in the small airways, the recording of closing volume has been considered an ideal test for early detection of airway disease. The use of the test is not as popular as it was earlier, however, because its reproducibility is not as good as that of conventional spirometry. Even if the recording of airway

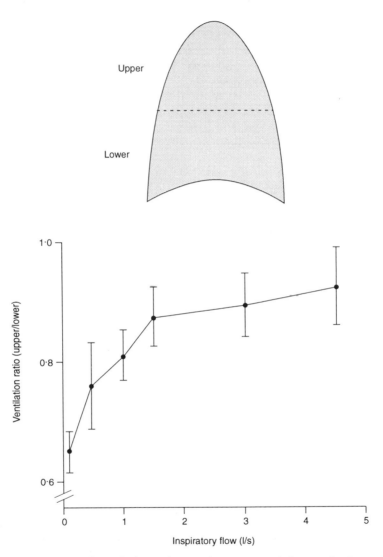

Fig 5.2 The ratio of ventilation going to the upper and that to the lower lung regions with a change in inspiratory flow. Note that distribution of ventilation to the lower lung regions is at a low flow rate (for an explanation, see Fig 5.1). This is replaced, however, by a more even distribution with increasing flow, as, for example, during exercise. This ensures more efficient use of the lung tissue and the alveolar–capillary membranes for gas transfer (provided that pulmonary blood flow shows a similar distribution pattern). (Redrawn from Bake et al.[5])

closure as a diagnostic and quantitative measure of lung disease may not have been as successful as hoped for, it should not obscure the fact that airway closure is a most important phenomenon, and its detection has taught us a lot about the physiological principles governing the distribution of ventilation.

As mentioned above, secretions, oedema, and spasm reduce the airway lumen. This affects gas distribution as well, decreasing or eliminating ventilation in regions that are affected by airway obstruction, and increasing it in other, less obstructed, areas.

Voluntary efforts to change gas distribution

Can the distribution of ventilation be voluntarily altered? This question is certainly frequently asked by physiotherapists as well as physicians when faced with a hypoxaemic patient struggling for air. It has been assumed that, if the diaphragm is preferentially used ("abdominal breathing"), then basal lung regions would be better ventilated, and it would also open up closed regions and improve aeration. There is, however, little proof that it

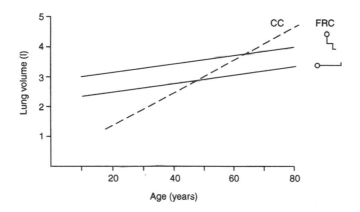

Fig 5.3   Resting lung volume (FRC), upright and supine, and closing capacity (CC, unaffected by body positions) at different ages in healthy subjects. Note the lower FRC, by about 0·7–0·8 l, in the supine position (an effect of the cranial displacement of the diaphragm by the abdominal organs). As can be seen, there is also a slight increase in FRC with age, at constant height and weight. This is an effect of the loss of elastic tissue with ageing. Finally, observe the more rapid increase in CC with age. This results in airway closure above the FRC in upright patients aged 65–70 years or more. In the supine position, airways may already close during breathing at ages of 45–50 years! This relationship between CC and FRC is a probable explanation for the decreasing oxygenation of blood with age. The curves are based on pooled data from different studies. See the literature.[6 7]

does. On the contrary, when the distribution of inspired air has been studied using an isotope technique, it has been exactly the same from the apex to the base of the lung, whether mainly the rib cage or the diaphragm has been allowed to move.[8] This does not exclude an effect at a smaller level that can be detected by the technique used, particularly in the alveoli lining the chest wall. The importance of such a possible effect will, however, be less.

There are two other approaches that may affect gas distribution: (1) varying the inspiratory airflow, and (2) varying the depth of inspiration. The first has already been discussed at some length above, and it is only mentioned that, the slower the inspiratory flow, the more air goes to dependent lung regions. In the second approach, the deeper the inspiration, the more the closed airways are opened, and this occurs primarily in dependent lung regions. Thus, a slow and deep inspiration favours lower, dependent lung regions, which is of value, because perfusion of the lung is greater in the lower regions—an effect of gravity, as discussed later. Increased ventilation of dependent regions accordingly improves gas exchange.

Another aspect of deliberately modifying ventilation is to expire against a resistance, for example, against half closed lips ("pursed lips breathing"). Doing this, a patient with chronic obstructive disease frequently experiences that his or her breathing becomes easier. Devices are also available to breathe out using that technique as a resistance. It has often been suggested that this builds up a higher pressure inside the airway, preventing it from closing during expiration and is the reason why breathing is more comfortable. Thus, the device "stabilises" the airway and facilitates expiration.[9] Although the result may be the desired one, the explanation is wrong. The higher airway pressure can be generated only by increasing the expiratory effort and this increases the pleural pressure to the same extent as the airway pressure. The pressure drop across the airway wall is the same as it would be without expiratory resistance, and this does not make the airway more stable. What may explain the beneficial result is that the expiratory resistance increases the lung volume and slows down expiration. The lung volume increase is the only way of increasing transpulmonary and transairway pressure and this stabilises the airway. Simultaneously, there is a general increase in airway calibre which reduces the resistance further, as discussed above. The slowed expiration reduces the pressure drop from the alveoli towards the mouth, because lower flow requires less driving pressure. By this means, the point along the airway tree at which pressure inside the airway has dropped to below that outside the airway (equal to pleural pressure) is moved towards the mouth. Thus, slow expiratory flow may make it possible to move the "equal pressure point", where inside and outside airway pressures are equal, up to the larger airways or the mouth and this prevents floppy airways from collapsing[10] (Fig 5.4).

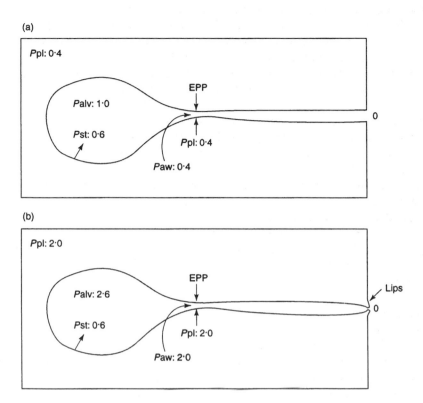

Fig 5.4 A schematic drawing of the "equal pressure point" (EPP) concept and dynamic compression of airways. (a) Normal breathing: a slightly forced expiration during otherwise normal conditions. By the application of some expiratory muscle effort pleural pressure (Ppl) is positive—0·4 kPa (4 cm H_2O). The elastic recoil pressure (Pst) of the alveoli (0·6 kPa) and the pleural pressure add together to yield the intra-alveolar pressure (Palv = 1·0 kPa). This causes an expiratory flow. At some point downstream, the airway pressure (Paw) has dropped by 0·6 kPa, so that intraluminal pressure and pleural, extraluminal pressure are the same. This is the EPP. From this point to the mouth, intraluminal airway pressure is lower than surrounding, extraluminal pressure and the airway may be compressed. (b) An attempt to stabilise the airway by so called "pursed lips" breathing. The increased resistance to expiratory flow requires an increased expiratory effort to maintain airflow. Thus, pleural pressure is increased compared with the normal conditions in (a) (Ppl = 2·0 kPa). Alveolar elastic recoil pressure (Pst) is the same as in (a), provided that the lung volume is the same. If expiratory flow is of the same magnitude as during normal breathing, pressure along the airway falls to the same extent as during normal breathing. Thus, the EPP will have the same location as during normal breathing and no stabilisation of the airway has been achieved. The only way of moving the EPP towards the mouth and to less collapsible airways is (1) by raising the alveolar recoil pressure (Pst) by an increase in lung volume, or (2) by lowering expiratory flow rate so that the pressure drop along the airway tree is slowed down.

29

1 Milic-Emili J, Henderson JAM, Dolovich MB, Trop D, Kaneko K. Regional distribution of inspired gas in the lung. *J Appl Physiol* 1966;**21**:749–59.
2 Guy HJ, Prisk GK, Elliott AR, Deutschman RA III, West JB. Inhomogeneity of pulmonary ventilation during sustained microgravity as determined by single-breath washouts. *J Appl Physiol* 1994;**76**:1719–29.
3 Crawford AB, Makowska M, Paiva M, Engel LA. Convection- and diffusion-dependent ventilation maldistribution in normal subjects. *J Appl Physiol* 1985;**59**:838–46.
4 Ganesan S, Lai-Fook SJ. Finite element analysis of regional lung expansion in prone and supine positions: effect of heart weight and diaphragmatic compliance. *Physiologist* 1989;**32**:191.
5 Bake B, Wood L, Murphy B, Macklem PT, Milic-Emili J. Effect of inspiratory flow rate on regional distribution of inspired gas. *J Appl Physiol* 1974;**37**:8–17.
6 Leblanc P, Ruff F, Milic Emili J. Effects of age and body position on "airway closure" in man. *J Appl Physiol* 1970;**28**:448–51.
7 McCarthy DS, Spencer R, Greene R, Milic-Emili J. Measurement of "closing volume" as a simple and sensitive test for early detection of small airway disease. *Am J Med* 1972;**52**:747–53.
8 Bake B, Fugl-Meyer AR, Grimby G. Breathing pattern and regional ventilation distribution in tetraplegic patients and in normal subjects. *Clin Sci* 1972;**42**:117.
9 Jones NL. Physical therapy—present state of the art. *Am Rev Respir Dis* 1974;**110**:132–6.
10 Mead J, Turner J, Macklem PT, Little JB. Significance of the relationship between lung recoil and maximum respiratory flow. *J Appl Physiol* 1967;**22**:95–108.

6:   Diffusion of gas

Diffusion of gas occurs both in the airways and across the alveolar–capillary membranes and is dealt with in this chapter.

Diffusion in airways and alveoli

Airflow is convective in the larger and medium sized airways, down to about the fourteenth generation. Airways at this level start to become tapered into alveoli and participate in gas exchange with pulmonary blood. In the later generations of airways, from the fifteenth to the twenty third, the total cross sectional area of the airway tree grows rapidly, from 2·5 cm^2 in the trachea, 70 cm^2 in the fourteenth generation entering the acinus, to 0·8 m^2 in the twenty third generation.[1] The total alveolar surface is about 140 m^2. Airflow velocity decreases at the same rate as the area increases. For an ordinary breath, the average velocity of air in the trachea is about 0·7 m/s, but at the alveolar surface it is no higher than 0·001 mm/s. This is much slower than the diffusion rate of O_2 and CO_2 in the airway tree and the alveoli. Transport of O_2 and CO_2 is therefore by diffusion in the peripheral airways and in the alveoli, not by convective flow. Carbon dioxide can be detected in the mouth after a few seconds of breath-hold. This is the result, however, not only of diffusion but also of convection, brought about by the beating heart, which acts as a mixing pump. Even in the absence of heart beats, CO_2 appears within seconds at the airway opening. This rapid diffusion has an implication when measuring dead space by recording the expiratory CO_2 curve—an inspiratory breath-hold reducing the measured dead space down to zero, if the breath is kept just for a few seconds.

It has often been discussed whether gas mixing is complete in the alveoli of a normal lung during normal breathing, or if there are concentration gradients, often called "stratified inhomogeneity". Many consider alveolar concentrations to be homogeneous. If the alveolar dimensions grow, however, by expansion or confluence of several alveoli, as in emphysema, the diffusion distance can be too large to allow complete mixing of inspired air and alveolar gas during ordinary breathing. This causes stratified inhomogeneity of respiratory gas concentrations within the alveolar unit, and has an impeding effect on gas exchange, similar to the uneven distribution of ventilation by other means.[2]

Diffusion across alveolar–capillary membranes

Oxygen diffuses passively from the alveolar gas phase into the plasma and to the red cells, where it binds to the haemoglobin. Carbon dioxide diffuses in the opposite direction, from the plasma to the alveoli. The amount that can diffuse over the membranes for a given period of time is determined by:[3]

1 The surface area available for diffusion
2 The thickness of the membranes
3 The pressure difference for the gas across the barrier
4 The molecular weight of the gas
5 The solubility of the gas in the tissues it has to traverse.

These factors are discussed below.

Surface area

The lung volume is obviously of importance. The smaller the lung, the less the overall diffusion. To this should be added that the lung surface (or its major extent) can be used only for diffusion if there is circulating blood on the capillary side. Thus, pulmonary capillary blood volume is an important determinant of diffusion. The relative influence of the membrane area and characteristics, and that of capillary blood volume, can also be analysed separately, as discussed in Part III.

Membrane thickness

The thicker the membrane, the longer the diffusion distance and the lower the diffusion capacity. In addition, if the solubility of the gas is lowered by thickening of the membrane, diffusion is impeded even more (see below).

Pressure gradient

The larger the difference in O_2 or CO_2 tensions between the gas phase in the alveolus and the plasma in the capillary, the greater the diffusion. The mixed venous blood entering the pulmonary capillary has a Po_2 of 5·3 kPa (40 mm Hg) and the alveolar Po_2 is about 13·3 kPa (100 mm Hg), creating a driving pressure of 8 kPa (60 mm Hg). When blood flows in the capillary, it takes up O_2 (and delivers CO_2), but as O_2 pressure builds up in the capillary blood, the diffusion rate slows down and becomes zero when pressure is equilibrated over the alveolar–capillary wall (Fig 6.1). In the normal lung at low cardiac output, equilibrium has been reached within 25–30% of the capillary distance, and no gas transfer takes place in the remaining capillary. When cardiac output is increased, as during exercise, blood passes faster through the capillary and a longer length of capillary is required before equilibrium can be reached, equilibration time being much the same as during resting conditions (a lower venous P_{O_2} speeds up diffusion at the start). Thickened alveolar–capillary membranes prolong the equilibration process with the possibility of developing hypoxaemia. This is dealt with in more detail in chapter 18.

It should also be mentioned that most of the O_2 that dissolves in plasma, diffuses into the red cell and binds to the haemoglobin: 1 g haemoglobin can bind 1·36 ml O_2 (combining factors between 1·34 and 1·39 are used). This means that 1 l of blood with a haemoglobin of 150 g/l can bind 204 ml O_2, if fully saturated. With a saturation of 98%, which is normally achieved in arterial blood, the haemoglobin bound O_2 amounts to 200 ml/l blood. This should be compared with the 3 ml O_2 that is physically dissolved in 1 l blood with a P_{aO_2} of 13·3 kPa (100 mm Hg). The haemoglobin bound O_2 creates no pressure in the plasma. This is important, because it allows much more O_2 to diffuse over the membranes before pressure equilibration is reached. Anaemia reduces, and polycythaemia increases, the diffusion capacity.

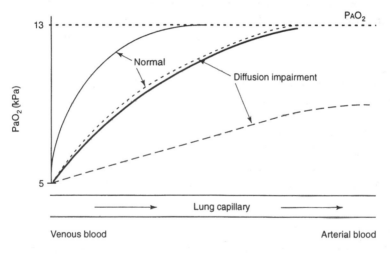

Fig 6.1 Oxygenation of pulmonary capillary blood at rest (—) and during exercise (- - -) in a normal subject and in a patient with fibrotic lung disease with diffusion impairment. In the normal subject there is a rapid equilibration of the oxygen tension in capillary blood with that in alveolar gas. This has been achieved within one third of the capillary distance. During exercise, however, most of the capillary distance must be used to reach equilibration between alveolar and pulmonary capillary oxygen tensions. This is an effect of the shorter transit time of red blood cells resulting from the increased cardiac output. Distension and recruitment of pulmonary capillaries may to some extent offset the effect of raised cardiac output on the velocity of the blood through the capillaries. With a diffusion impairment, equilibration takes longer, but full equilibration may still be reached at rest. With increased blood velocity during exercise, however, the equilibration of oxygen may be far from complete at the end of the pulmonary capillary, causing desaturation of arterial blood that may sometimes be severe.

33

Molecular weight

The diffusion coefficient of a gas is inversely related to the square root of the molecular weight of the gas. Thus, the larger the molecule, the more difficult it is for it to traverse a membrane. Oxygen is a relatively light gas with a molecular weight of 32. Carbon dioxide is heavier with a molecular weight of 44, and should therefore be more limited in its diffusion than O_2. Taking the square root of the weights reduces the difference between the gases, however, and, in practice, CO_2 is much more diffusible than O_2, as explained below.

Solubility

The diffusion process is linearly related to tissue solubility of the gas. The solubility is usually set equal to that of gas in water: CO_2 is almost 30 times more soluble in water than O_2, and so it diffuses more than 20 times faster (the net effect of all factors gone through here).[3] In practice, this means that there is no lung disease, compatible with life, that causes a measurable diffusion impairment for CO_2.

1 Haefeli-Bleuer B, Weibel ER. Morphometry of the human pulmonary acinus. *Anat Rec* 1988;**220**:401–14.
2 Adaro F, Piiper J. Limiting role of stratification in alveolar exchange of oxygen. *Respir Physiol* 1976;**26**:195–206.
3 West JB. *Respiratory physiology – the essentials*, 4th edn. Baltimore, MD: Williams & Wilkins, 1990: 21–30.

7: Pulmonary perfusion

Low pressure system

The pulmonary circulation is a low pressure system, compared with the systemic circulation. A pulmonary artery pressure (typically, systolic 20 mm Hg and diastolic 8 mm Hg) is about six to ten times lower than in the systemic artery. The lower pressure is achieved by the larger vascular diameter and shorter length of the pulmonary vessels, compared with the systemic ones. In particular, a large vascular lumen decreases the demand on driving pressure. According to Poiseuille's law, a decrease in vascular radius reduces the pressure demand by an exponent of four to maintain a certain flow, if flow is linear. With turbulent flow, the dependence on vascular dimensions will be even higher. As a consequence of the lower resistance, pulmonary capillary blood flow is pulsatile, contrary to the steady flow in systemic capillaries.[1] Another, presumably more important, consequence of the low pressure is that the capillary and alveolar walls can be made very thin without causing any plasma leakage, and this facilitates diffusion of O_2 and CO_2. A sudden increase in pulmonary artery pressure to a mean of over 30 mm Hg causes effusion of plasma into the interstitial and alveolar spaces, that is, lung oedema. A slower increase in pressure, over months or years, stimulates the growth of the vascular smooth muscles ("vascular remodelling") with thickening of the vascular wall.[2] Oedema is prevented more effectively, despite even severe pulmonary hypertension, but at the cost of impaired diffusion capacity.

Distribution of lung blood flow

The blood flow through the lung is governed by the driving pressure and the vascular resistance. If these are unevenly distributed, then perfusion may also be uneven, which seems to be the case. What the perfusion distribution looks like, and the mechanisms behind it, have, however, become a subject of much debate during recent years. Thus, the previously generally accepted explanation of a gravitational orientation of perfusion, as demonstrated in the pioneering work by Permutt and by West and co-workers,[3] has recently been challenged by others who propose a "fractal" distribution with gravity playing only a minor role.[4] Here, the "gravitational" concept is dealt with first, and then the "fractal" one.

Gravitational distribution of lung blood flow

Pulmonary artery pressure increases down the lung, an effect of the hydrostatic pressure that builds up on the way from the top to the bottom of the lung. This pressure increases by 1 cm H_2O/cm distance down the lung (or 0·74 mm Hg/cm vertical distance—blood has a density close to 1, or 1·04). This causes a pressure difference in the pulmonary arterial vessels, between the apex and the base, of some 11–15 mm Hg, depending on the height of the lung. There is thus less driving pressure at the top of the lung. As the mean pulmonary artery pressure is about 12 mm Hg at the level of the heart, it may approach zero in the apex of the lung in the upright position. Moreover, if alveolar pressure is increased, as during positive pressure ventilation, it may exceed that in the pulmonary artery and compress the pulmonary capillaries. No blood then flows through the vessels. This part of the lung is called zone I, according to the nomenclature introduced by West and associates[3] (see Fig 5.1). If arterial pressure and capillary pressure exceed alveolar pressure, as they do further down the lung because of the addition of hydrostatic pressure, blood flow is established. The perfusion pressure is arterial pressure minus alveolar pressure, as long as alveolar pressure exceeds that of the pulmonary veins. This is different from the systemic circulation, where perfusion pressure is arterial pressure minus venous pressure. Moreover, the increasing pulmonary arterial pressure down the lung and the constant alveolar pressure increase the perfusion pressure down this part of the lung, called zone II, with the consequent increase in blood flow. Further down the lung, both arterial and venous pressures exceed pressure in the alveoli, so that perfusion pressure is arterial pressure minus venous pressure. This part of the lung is called zone III. As both arterial and venous pressures increase to the same extent down through zone III, with hydrostatic pressure adding to both sides, perfusion pressure does not increase. Perfusion does increase downwards, although it may be less than the increase in zone II. The explanation proposed is that the increasing vascular pressure dilates the vessels down the lung, and by this means reduces the vascular resistance.[3]

A few years after these initial observations, it was noticed that blood flow decreased in the bottom of the lung, so zone IV was added to the model of lung perfusion.[3] This called for a new explanation, which suggested that an increasing interstitial pressure down the lung pressed on the extra-alveolar vessels and made them narrower. The vertical distribution of blood flow could, accordingly, be explained by the influence of gravitation on vascular, alveolar, and interstitial pressures.

The homogeneity of blood flow distribution has also been tested during zero gravity or microgravity shuttle flights with the NASA Space Laboratory. Using indirect techniques, based on an analysis of the variation of expired gas concentrations that are synchronous with the heart beats ("cardiogenic oscillations"), more uniform lung blood flow distribution was recorded.[4]

Non-gravitational inhomogeneity of blood flow distribution

In experiments with dogs, groups at the Mayo Clinic and subsequently in Seattle noticed that the vertical lung blood flow distribution was rather even, and did not change when position was altered between supine and prone.[5] This made the Seattle group conclude that gravity was of minor importance in determining perfusion distribution. The same group also showed that perfusion at a given vertical level is unevenly distributed on that horizontal plane, with an inhomogeneity that far exceeded that in the vertical direction. In carefully repeated experiments, they managed to reproduce the same pattern of inhomogeneity. This suggests that there are morphological and/or functional differences between lung vessels which also, and perhaps more importantly than gravity, determine blood flow distribution. In their hypothesis, they postulate that blood flow in the lung varies between lung regions, and that the variation becomes larger the smaller the lung unit under study. This could explain the failure to find a non-gravitational inhomogeneity of blood flow in early studies, with poorer resolution of the techniques used.

Other groups have also made observations suggesting an uneven distribution of blood flow, which cannot be explained by gravity, with more blood going to the core of the lung and less to the periphery.[6] A longer distance to the peripheral bed was offered as an explanation, causing larger vascular resistance to the periphery. Others, however, found less difference between central and peripheral lung regions. The application of a positive end expiratory pressure (PEEP) in anaesthetised and mechanically ventilated dogs forced perfusion of the lung towards the periphery.[7] As always, the reliability of the techniques used is critical. It seems as if the spatial distribution of blood flow as measured by single photon emission computed tomography (SPECT) has reconstruction artefacts, a technique that has been used in some studies. Still others have used microsphere techniques and have measured the distribution in excised lungs. Although it may have other limitations, one could dare to conclude that enough evidence has been accumulated to believe in a non-gravitational inhomogeneity of lung perfusion.

Synopsis

Despite the rather hard stands taken for and against the "gravitational" and "fractal" concepts, it must be possible for both to exist simultaneously. Some of the disagreement may result from the fact that different species have been studied, including humans, and that differences exist in their habitual body position. Thus, vascular resistance seems to be lower in dorsal regions of horse lungs, compared with the anterior part.[8] It seems reasonable that, in an animal that is standing or resting on its four limbs most of the time, the vascular tree has adjusted to that position and, by increasing its resistance in anterior parts, made blood flow more evenly distributed. It may be that humans have a lung blood flow distribution that is more dependent on gravity than in many other species. If so, it may be an effect of a more varied body positioning which has never favoured the development of interlobar or other anatomically related differences in lung vascular resistance. Finally, what causes the large variation in the pulmonary microcirculation remains to be found, and also to what extent it affects gas exchange.

Hypoxic pulmonary vasoconstriction

It was noticed at the turn of century that hypoxia affects the pulmonary vasculature; this was rediscovered and studied in more detail in 1946.[9] Hypoxic pulmonary vasoconstriction (HPV) seems to be a compensatory mechanism, aimed at reducing blood flow in hypoxic lung regions. The major stimulus for HPV is a low alveolar O_2 tension, whether caused by hypoventilation or breathing of a gas with a low Po_2. The stimulus of mixed venous Po_2 is much weaker.[10] The strength of the constriction is also dependent on the size of the lung segment exposed to the hypoxia, being stronger the smaller the region. Thus, in humans studied during intravenous anaesthesia, assumed not to affect HPV, one lung hypoxia with 8% and 4% O_2 during contralateral hyperoxia (fractional concentration of inspired O_2, $Fo_2 = 1.0$) caused a blood flow diversion away from the hypoxic to the other, hyperoxic, lung, from 52% to 40%, and 30% of cardiac output.[11] There are species differences so that results in one kind of animal cannot be translated into another, or into humans. Pigs and cattle have highly developed HPV.[12] It is of interest that these animals have no collateral ventilation (ventilation between neighbouring alveoli via pores in the alveolar walls, or via interbronchial channels), so their only way of compensating for a regional decrease in ventilation is to reduce perfusion of that area in order to maintain a normal $\dot{V}/\dot{Q}$ match. On the other hand, global hypoxia can be detrimental to them, as seen when cattle were moved across the high plains during the colonisation of North America. They developed pulmonary hypertension which caused pulmonary oedema and even right heart failure; this has hardly been seen in other species.

Humans may also develop pulmonary hypertension and pulmonary oedema at high altitude.[13] Chronic lung disease with hypoxaemia also causes HPV, but the slow progress of the disease allows time for remodelling of the pulmonary vascular wall, which thickens to prevent oedema formation.[2]

1 Harris P, Heath D. *The human pulmonary circulation*. New York: Churchill Livingstone, 1986.
2 Wagenvoort CA, Wagenvoort N. Pulmonary vascular bed. Normal anatomy and response to disease. In: Moser KM, ed. *Pulmonary vascular disease*. New York: Marcel Dekker, 1979: 1–109.
3 West JB. Blood flow. In: West JB, ed. *Regional differences in the lung*. New York: Academic Press, 1977: 85–165.
4 Prisk GK, Guy HJ, Elliott AR, West JB. Inhomogeneity of pulmonary perfusion during sustained microgravity on SLS-1. *J Appl Physiol* 1994;76:1730–8.
5 Glenny RW, Lamm WJ, Albert RK, Robertson HT. Gravity is a minor determinant of pulmonary blood flow distribution. *J Appl Physiol* 1991;71:620–9.
6 Hakim TS, Lisbona R, Dean GW. Gravity-independent inequality in pulmonary blood flow in humans. *J Appl Physiol* 1987;63:1114–21.
7 Hedenstierna G, White F, Wagner PD. Spatial distribution of pulmonary blood flow in the dog with PEEP ventilation. *J Appl Physiol* 1979;47:938–46.
8 Hlastala MP, Bernard SL, Erickson HH, Fedde MR, Gaughan EM, McMurpy R, et al. Pulmonary blood flow distribution in standing horses is not determined by gravity. *J Appl Physiol* 1996;81:1051–61.
9 von Euler US, Liljestrand G. Observations on the pulmonary arterial blood pressure in cat. *Acta Physiol Scand* 1946;12:310–20.
10 Marshall BE. Effects of anesthetics on pulmonary gas exchange. In: Stanley TH, Sperry RJ, eds. *Anesthesia and the lung*. London: Kluwer Academic Press, 1989: 117–25.
11 Hambraeus-Jonzon K, Bindslev L, Jolin Mellgård Å, Hedenstierna G. Hypoxic pulmonary vasoconstriction in human lungs. *Anesthesiology* 1997;86:308–15.
12 Tucker AO, McMurtry IF, Reeves JT, Alexander AF, Will DH, Grover RF. Lung vascular smooth muscle as a determinant of pulmonary hypertension at high altitude. *Am J Physiol* 1975;228:762–7.
13 Antezana G, Leguia G, Guzman AM, Coudert J, Spielvogel H. Hemodynamic study of high altitude pulmonary edema (12,200 ft). In: Bredel W, Zink RA, eds. *High altitude physiology and medicine*. New York: Springer Verlag, 1982: 232–41.

8: Causes of hypoxaemia and hypercapnia

In the previous chapters we have discussed ventilation, gas distribution, and the respiratory mechanics that govern distribution, diffusion, and pulmonary perfusion. All these components of lung function can affect the oxygenation of blood, and all except diffusion can also measurably affect CO_2 elimination. The different mechanisms behind hypoxaemia and CO_2 retention, or hypercapnia or hypercarbia, have been touched on, but are analysed in more detail here.

Causes of hypoxaemia can suitably be divided into:

1 Hypoventilation
2 Ventilation–perfusion ($\dot{V}_A/\dot{Q}$) mismatch
3 Diffusion impairment
4 Right-to-left shunt.

Hypercapnia can be caused by hypoventilation, $\dot{V}_A/\dot{Q}$ mismatch, and shunt, although in practice hypoventilation is the only one of real importance (Tables 8.1 and 8.2).

Hypoventilation

If ventilation is low in proportion to the metabolic demand, the elimination of CO_2 will be inadequate, and CO_2 accumulates in the alveoli,

Table 8.1   Causes of hypoxaemia

Disturbance	P_{aO_2} (air) at rest	P_{aO_2} (O_2) at rest	P_{aO_2} (air) on exercise (compared with rest)	P_{aCO_2}
Hypoventilation	Reduced	Normal	No change or further decrease	Increased
$\dot{V}_A/\dot{Q}$ mismatch	Reduced	Normal	No or minor increase or decrease	Normal
Shunt	Reduced	Reduced	No change or further decrease	Normal
Diffusion impairment	Reduced	Normal	Small to large decrease	Normall

Table 8.2   Mechanisms of hypoxaemia in different lung disorders

Disorder	Hypoventilation	Diffusion impairment	$\dot{V}_A/\dot{Q}$ mismatch	Shunt
Chronic bronchitis	(+)	−	+ +	−
Emphysema	+	+ +	+ + +	−
Asthma	−	−	+ +	−
Fibrosis	−	+ +	+	+
Pneumonia	−	−	+	+ +
Atelectasis	−	−	−	+ +
Pulmonary oedema	−	+	+	+ +
Pulmonary emboli	−	−	+ +	+
ARDS	−	−	+	+ + +

blood, and other body tissues. Hypoventilation is often defined as a ventilation that results in a $P_{a_{CO_2}}$ (arterial CO_2 tension) above 6 kPa (45 mm Hg). With this definition, hypoventilation can be present even when minute ventilation is high, if the metabolic demand or the dead space ventilation is increased more than minute ventilation. An example of increased metabolic demand is the rise in $P_{a_{CO_2}}$ that can be seen in athletes during maximum physical exercise, but more seldom in normally fit subjects, in whom cardiac function limits performance before maximum ventilation has been reached. This may be considered of minor importance for a clinician, but can be a top priority in the super-athlete, struggling for an Olympic medal (this book is being drafted in the shade of the summer Olympics 1996). Examples of increased dead space ventilation are the large increases in dead space that can be seen in chronic pulmonary embolism (maintained ventilation of non-perfused lung units), and in chronic bronchitis and emphysema (redistribution of ventilation away from regions with high airway resistance to regions with lower resistance, so that they become ventilated well in excess of their perfusion).[1] These patients mostly have large minute ventilations, even the bronchitic patient who is often accused of hypoventilating (the "blue bloater"). During exercise, the patient with severe obstructive lung disease may show increasing CO_2 tension in blood, a reasonable effect of heavy respiratory work and poor ventilation–perfusion matching.[2]

The increased $P_{A_{CO_2}}$ (alveolar CO_2 tension) reduces the space available for O_2 in the alveoli. The $P_{A_{O_2}}$ can be estimated by the alveolar gas equation, shown in full in the box in chapter 18 (page 142). A simplified form is deducted here. Thus, assuming a normal respiratory exchange ratio, $P_{A_{O_2}}$ can be calculated as:

$$P_{A_{O_2}} = P_{I_{O_2}} - [1 \cdot 25 \times P_{A_{CO_2}}].$$

The factor $1 \cdot 25$ is correct if the respiratory exchange ratio is $0 \cdot 8$ and this can be reasonably assumed under resting conditions. $P_{A_{CO_2}}$ can be assumed to equal Pa_{CO_2}. Thus, with a PI_{O_2} of 19·9 kPa (149 mm Hg) and a Pa_{CO_2} of 5·3 kPa (40 mm Hg), PA_{O_2} is 13·2 kPa (99 mm Hg), and, during hypoventilation with a Pa_{CO_2} of 8 kPa (60 mm Hg), PA_{CO_2} is 9·9 kPa (74 mm Hg). This gives the highest possible Pa_{O_2} that can exist at that level of alveolar ventilation. Thus, whether a low Pa_{O_2} can be explained by hypoventilation can be tested easily by this simple formula. If there is a gap between the estimated PA_{O_2} and the measured Pa_{O_2}, another or additional cause of hypoxaemia must be sought. It is also obvious that the decrease in Pa_{O_2} caused by hypoventilation is easily overcome by increasing the PI_{O_2} (which, on the other hand, may decrease the stimulus to breath and cause further retention of CO_2).

Ventilation–perfusion mismatch

For optimum gas exchange, ventilation and perfusion must match each other in all lung regions. At rest both ventilation and perfusion increase down the lung. Perfusion increases more than ventilation, the difference between the uppermost and lowermost 5 cm segments being three times for ventilation and ten times for perfusion. This results in a mean alveolar ventilation–perfusion ratio ($\dot{V}A/\dot{Q}$) of about 1, somewhere in the middle of the lung, and a range of $\dot{V}A/\dot{Q}$ ratios from 0·5 in the bottom of the lung to 5 in non-dependent regions (Fig 8.1). With exercise, the spatial distribution of ventilation and blood flow become more even, as discussed earlier. This makes more efficient use of the alveolar–capillary surface for gas transfer, and increases the gas exchanging capacity. It also reduces the "normal" $\dot{V}A/\dot{Q}$ mismatch.[1]

If ventilation and perfusion are not matched, gas exchange will be affected. The most common cause of oxygenation impairment is indeed $\dot{V}A/\dot{Q}$ mismatch. Low $\dot{V}A/\dot{Q}$ ratio will impede oxygenation because ventilation is too small to oxygenate the blood fully. The degree of impairment is dependent on the degree of mismatch, and already the normally existing lung regions with $\dot{V}A/\dot{Q}$ ratios between 0·5 and 1 are unable to saturate the blood completely. Thus Pa_{O_2} is seldom equal to PA_{O_2}, but a difference (A–aP_{O_2}) exists, of about 0·4–0·7 kPa (3–5 mm Hg), in the normal lung. With more $\dot{V}A/\dot{Q}$ mismatch, A–aP_{O_2} is increased further. The $\dot{V}A/\dot{Q}$ mismatch can account for all the hypoxaemia seen in a severely obstructive patient.[3] Shunt, which is often claimed to exist in chronic obstructive pulmonary disease (COPD), is mostly absent when analysed with more sophisticated techniques, such as multiple inert gas elimination (see chapter 19). Indeed, shunt in an obstructive patient should be considered to signal a complicating factor in the disease (Fig 8.2).

In severe asthma it is common to see a distinct mode of low $\dot{V}A/\dot{Q}$ ratios when using the multiple inert gas elimination technique.[4] Thus, a bimodal distribution of $\dot{V}A/\dot{Q}$ ratios can be seen (Fig 8.3). The explanation is

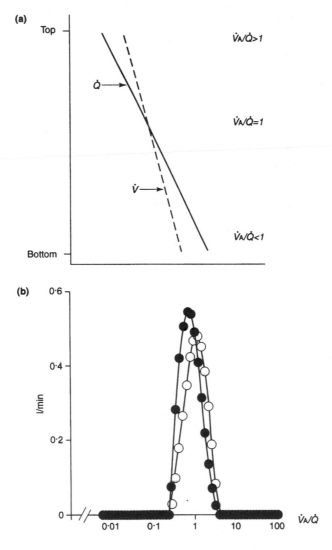

Fig 8.1 A schematic drawing of (a) the vertical distributions of ventilation ($\dot{V}$) and blood flow through the lung ($\dot{Q}$) and (b) the resulting ventilation–perfusion distribution ($\dot{V}A/\dot{Q}$). Note the moderate increase in ventilation (o) down the lung and the faster increase in perfusion (●). The $\dot{V}A/\dot{Q}$ distribution is centred upon a ratio of 1, corresponding to the intersection of the two ventilation and perfusion distribution curves. The slightly larger ventilation than perfusion in the upper lung regions contributes to the high $\dot{V}A/\dot{Q}$ ratios (> 1), whereas the larger perfusion than ventilation in the lower part of the lung is the cause of the lower $\dot{V}A/\dot{Q}$ ratios (< 1). For further details about the assessment of ventilation–perfusion ratios, see chapter 19.

43

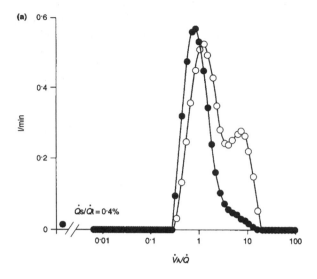

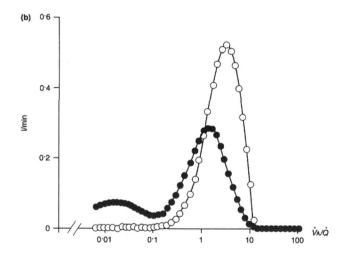

Fig 8.2 Examples of impaired matching of ventilation and lung blood flow in chronic obstructive lung disease. (○, ventilation; ●, perfusion). (a) The $\dot{V}_A/\dot{Q}$ distribution in a patient referred to as a "pink puffer". Note the broader $\dot{V}_A/\dot{Q}$ distribution compared with that in Fig 8.1. This is mainly the effect of the presence of ventilation of regions with high $\dot{V}_A/\dot{Q}$ ratios. This causes a dead space like effect. There is little of perfusion of poorly ventilated lung regions. There was also almost no shunt. The arterial oxygenation was good. (b) Another obstructed patient, categorised as a "blue bloater". Note the markedly wide $\dot{V}_A/\dot{Q}$ distribution with ventilation going to regions with relatively high $\dot{V}_A/\dot{Q}$ ratios and the considerable amount of perfusion to regions with low $\dot{V}_A/\dot{Q}$ ratios. These cause hypoxaemia despite the lack of a shunt. $\dot{Q}_s/\dot{Q}_t$ is the shunt fraction.

44

probably that alveoli behind completely obstructed airways (oedema, mucus plugging, spasm) can still be ventilated via alveolar pores and interbronchial communications—so called collateral ventilation. This may also explain why shunt is not normally seen in COPD (Fig 8.4). With standard techniques, however, such as calculation of shunt by the O_2 equation, low $\dot{V}A/\dot{Q}$ cannot be separated from shunt. The expression "venous admixture" should be used in that case.

It should be understood that airway obstructions are unevenly distributed over the lung, and a large variation in $\dot{V}A/\dot{Q}$ ratios can be seen in a single patient. Indeed, ventilation is redistributed from regions with high

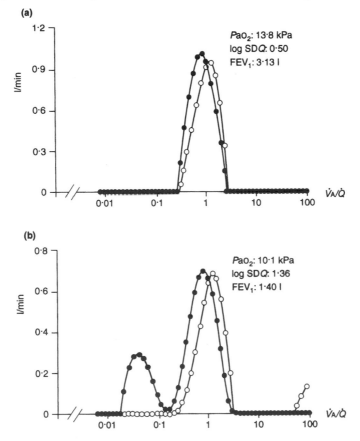

Fig 8.3 An example of $\dot{V}A/\dot{Q}$ distributions of a patient with allergic asthma. (a) The baseline data with an essential normal $\dot{V}A/\dot{Q}$ distribution as well as normal Pao_2 and FEV_1. (b) Half an hour after antigen provocation. Note the appearance of a distinct low $\dot{V}A/\dot{Q}$ mode and no shunt. FEV_1 was drastically reduced and Pao_2 was also lowered. A possible explanation for the distinct bimodal $\dot{V}A/\dot{Q}$ distribution in asthma is given in Fig 8.4. (From Lagerstrand et al,[10] with permission from the authors and the publisher.)

45

tissue itself becomes a limiting factor. The only way to increase the gas transfer would be to increase the available surface area for diffusion (which is why ventilation and blood flow are more evenly distributed in the lung during exercise), or the driving pressure across the membranes (increasing the P_{IO_2}, if sports rules would allow it; the mixed venous P_{O_2} is already down at 1·5–2·0 kPa (10–15 mm Hg) and can hardly be lowered any further), or the O_2 carrying capacity in blood for a given P_{O_2} (stimulating red cell production or increasing the haemoglobin content by other means, if permissible). In the normally trained subject, P_{aO_2} hardly drops at maximum performance, because the limiting factor is more likely to be the cardiac output or the performance of the exercising muscles.

There is still one more condition where even healthy lungs may exert a limitation on diffusion, and that is breathing low concentrations of oxygen, for example, atmospheric air at extreme altitude. Low P_{IO_2} lowers the pressure difference across the alveolar–capillary membranes so that pressure equilibration between alveoli and capillaries may not have time to take place. Although this is mostly a minor contribution to the lowered P_{aO_2}, the major part is caused by the low P_{AO_2} itself. One example is the P_{aO_2} that can be anticipated at the summit of Mount Everest. Barometric pressure is around 250 mm Hg, resulting in a P_{IO_2} of no more than 5·72 kPa (43 mm Hg). Getting to the top requires extreme exercise, so the respiratory exchange ratio can be set at 1. P_{AO_2} can then be set to 5·72 kPa (43 mm Hg) minus P_{aCO_2}:

$$P_{AO_2} = 5·72 - P_{aCO_2} \text{ kPa}$$

or

$$P_{AO_2} = 43 - P_{aCO_2} \text{ mm Hg.}$$

Expired gas samples were collected during an expedition in 1981 and showed an astonishingly low end tidal P_{CO_2} of about 1 kPa (7–8 mm Hg).[8] This gave a P_{AO_2} of 4·7–4·8 kPa (35–36 mm Hg). At that partial pressure, diffusion limitation will occur that further lowers P_{aO_2}, down to below or around 4 kPa (30 mm Hg). If the extreme hyperventilation cannot be maintained, P_{aO_2} may drop to a catastrophic level. Climbing the summit of Mount Everest without supplementary O_2 takes its toll—mental dysfunction with loss of memory, headache, and other signs of cerebral impairment are regularly noticed afterwards.

Right-to-left shunt

If blood passes through the lung without coming into contact with ventilated alveoli, the blood will not be oxygenated or release CO_2. This is a shunt and it lowers P_{aO_2} and increases, although less easily observed, P_{aCO_2}. A small shunt of 2–3% of cardiac output can be seen in the normal subject, caused by thebesian veins that drain the heart and empty into the left atrium. In pathological states, shunt may amount to anything between near normal to above 50% of cardiac output. Shunt may be considered an extreme of mismatch, with a $\dot{V}_A/\dot{Q}$ ratio of zero. There are, however, clear differences between the concepts of mismatch and shunt. First, the anatomical basis differs. Regions with low $\dot{V}_A/\dot{Q}$ ratios are caused by airway and vascular narrowing, reducing ventilation and blood flow in some regions and increasing them in others. Examples are obstructive lung disease and vascular disorders. Shunt is caused by the complete cessation of ventilation in a region, usually caused by collapse (atelectasis) or consolidation (pneumonia, oedema, obliterative processes). Contrary to what is normally said, asthma, bronchitis, and emphysema do not cause shunt.[3][4] If shunt is found, it indicates a complication. Second, the effect of "low $\dot{V}_A/\dot{Q}$" on oxygenation of blood can essentially be overcome by adding more O_2 to the inspired air. Even in a poorly ventilated lung unit, P_{AO_2} can be increased almost as much as in normal regions, the difference being caused by the higher P_{ACO_2} in the poorly ventilated units. The effect of a moderate shunt can be reduced, but not eliminated, by giving more oxygen, because the non-ventilated region cannot be reached by the inspired gas. Thus, shunt will always lower P_{aO_2} at any P_{IO_2}, compared with what would have been measured without a shunt. When the shunt increases to 25%, the rise in P_{aO_2} will be small; with a shunt of 30% or more, there is almost no effect of added O_2.[9] This is the net effect of mixing blood with normal pulmonary end capillary P_{O_2} and shunt blood with a mixed venous P_{O_2}. If the shunt blood is a large enough fraction of total lung blood flow, the additional O_2 that can be physically dissolved by the raised P_{IO_2} is so small as to be almost immeasurable. The shunt is said to be refractory.

In a few patients who develop severe pulmonary hypertension, marked hypoxaemia may ensue, which cannot be explained by diffusion impairment or any other impairment in the lung. In these patients, the explanation may be a right-to-left shunt that develops when right atrial pressure exceeds that of the left atrium and pushes up the flap covering the foramen ovale in the interatrial septum. Normally, the flap has grown together with the septal wall, but, in as many as 10% of the population, the flap is loose and pressed over the foramen ovale as long as the pressure is higher in the left atrium. As the pressures in the atria do not vary exactly in phase, the right atrial pressure can exceed that of the left atrium during a short moment of the cardiac cycle, causing a shunt just during a brief period of the heart beat. Moreover, any circumstance that elevates the vascular pressures, and more so in the pulmonary circulation, may induce shunting or increase it. This is the reason why exercise can cause a temporary shunt.

1 West JB. Ventilation–perfusion relationships. *Am Rev Respir Dis* 1977;**116**:919–43.
2 Cohn JE, Donoso HD. Exercise and intrapulmonary ventilation–perfusion relationships in

chronic obstructive airway disease. *Am Rev Respir Dis* 1967;**95**:1015–25.

3 Wagner PD, Dantzker DR, Dueck R, Clausen JL, West JB. Ventilation–perfusion inequality in chronic obstructive pulmonary disease. *J Clin Invest* 1977;**59**:203–16

4 Wagner PD, Hedenstierna G, Bylin G. Ventilation–perfusion inequality in chronic asthma. *Am Rev Respir Dis* 1987;**136**:605–12.

5 Jernudd-Wilhelmsson Y, Hörnblad Y, Hedenstierna G. Ventilation–perfusion relationships in interstitial lung disease. *Eur J Respir Dis* 1986;**68**:39–49.

6 Manier G, Castaing Y, Guenard H. Determinants of hypoxemia during the acute phase of pulmonary embolism in humans. *Am Rev Respir Dis* 1985;**132**:332–8.

7 Hammond MD, Gale GE, Kapitan KS, Ries A, Wagner PD. Pulmonary gas exchange in humans during exercise at sea level. *J Appl Physiol* 1986;**60**:1590–8.

8 West JB, Hackett PH, Maret KH, Milledge JS, Peters RM Jr, Pizzo CJ, Winslow RM. Pulmonary gas exchange on the summit of Mount Everest. *J Appl Physiol* 1983;**55**:678–87.

9 Benatar SR, Hewlett AM, Nunn JF. The use of iso-shunt lines for control of oxygen therapy. *Br J Anaesth* 1973;**45**:711–18.

10 Lagerstrand, L, Larsson K, Ihre E, Zetterström O, Hedenstierna G. Pulmonary gas exchange response following allergen challenge in patients with allergic asthma. *Eur Respir J* 1992;**5**:1176–83.

Part II

Anaesthesia and acute respiratory failure

Anaesthesia causes an impairment of pulmonary function, whether the patient is breathing spontaneously or is ventilated mechanically after muscle paralysis. Impaired oxygenation of blood occurs in most subjects who are anaesthetised.[1] It has therefore become routine to add oxygen to the inspired gas so that the inspired O_2 fraction (FIO_2) is maintained at around 0·3–0·4. Despite these measures, mild to moderate hypoxaemia, defined as an arterial oxygen saturation of between 85% and 90%, may occur in about half of all patients undergoing elective surgery, and can last from a few seconds to up to 30 min. About 20% of the patients may have severe hypoxaemia, that is, the O_2 saturation is below 81% for up to 5 min.[2] Lung function remains impaired postoperatively, and clinically significant pulmonary complications can be seen in from 1–2% after minor surgery to up to 20% after upper abdominal and thoracic surgery.[3]

During the past ten years, it has been shown that there are qualitative similarities between morphological aspects and dysfunctions of the normal lung during anaesthesia and the severely diseased lung in acute respiratory failure (ARF) or acute respiratory distress syndrome (ARDS).[4] The quantitative differences in morphological and physiological disturbances are large, but it may still be convenient to bring both conditions together in a presentation of the hallmarks of pulmonary dysfunction during anaesthesia and in ARF.

1 Hedenstierna G. Ventilation–perfusion relationships during anaesthesia. *Thorax* 1995;**50**:85–91.
2 Moller JT, Johannessen NW, Berg H, Espersen K, Larsen LE. Hypoxaemia during anaesthesia—an observer study. *Br J Anaesth* 1991;**66**:437–44.
3 Kroenke K, Lawrence VA, Theroux JF, Tuley MR, Hilsenbeck S. Postoperative complications after thoracic and major abdominal surgery in patients with and without obstructive lung disease. *Chest* 1993;**104**:1445–51.
4 Gattinoni L, Pesenti A, Bombino M, Baglione S, Rivolta M, Rossi F, et al. Relationships between lung computed tomographic density, gas exchange and PEEP in acute respiratory failure. *Anesthesiology* 1988;**69**:824–32.

9: Respiratory mechanics during anaesthesia

In this chapter, the effects of anaesthesia on the mechanical behaviour of the respiratory system are discussed, followed by the effects on the ventilation and perfusion distributions and subsequent effects on gas exchange. As will be seen, the changes in the mechanical behaviour of the respiratory system have a major impact on the gas exchanging capacity.

Compliance and resistance of the respiratory system

The static compliance in the total respiratory system (lungs and chest wall) is reduced by, on average, from 95 to 60 ml/cm H_2O during anaesthesia.[1] Several studies on lung compliance have been carried out during anaesthesia and the vast majority of studies indicate a decrease compared with the awake state (for example, static compliance fell from a mean of 187 ml/cm H_2O awake to 149 ml/cm H_2O during anaesthesia when data from several studies were pooled).[1] Rehder and co-workers analysed possible sources of reduced compliance during anaesthesia in their 1976 review.[2] They considered direct anaesthetic effects on the lung tissue rather unlikely, but were unable at that time to evaluate possible effects of airway closure and atelectasis. These two phenomena are discussed in more detail in this chapter.

There are also studies on the resistance of the total respiratory system and the lungs during anaesthesia, most of them showing a considerable increase during both spontaneous breathing and mechanical ventilation.[1 2] The studies on resistance during anaesthesia have, however, been hampered by different experimental conditions during the awake and anaesthetised situations. Thus, a study that enables comparison of resistance under both isovolume and isoflow conditions is still missing. The possibility remains that the increased lung resistance merely reflects a reduced FRC during anaesthesia which is discussed next.

Lung volume and patency of airways and alveoli

Functional residual capacity and chest wall

The resting lung volume, or functional residual capacity (FRC), is reduced during anaesthesia. The supine body position by itself reduces FRC by 0·7–0·8 litre compared with the upright position, so that the further decrease of 0·4–0·5 litre caused by the anaesthesia decreases the FRC to near the awake residual volume. The reduction in FRC occurs with spontaneous breathing and whether the anaesthetic is inhaled or given intravenously.[3] Muscle paralysis and mechanical ventilation cause no further decrease in FRC. The average reduction corresponds to around 20% of the awake FRC and may contribute to an altered distribution of ventilation and impaired oxygenation of blood, as discussed later.

The decrease in FRC can be expected to be accompanied by a decrease in the transverse thoracic area or a cranial shift of the diaphragm. Using computed tomography (CT) a decrease in the chest area has been demonstrated, whereas reports on the shape and position of the diaphragm differ (Fig 9.1). Several studies suggest that the diaphragm is moved cephalad during anaesthesia, and so contributes to the decrease in FRC. A cephalad shift of the diaphragm may be explained by loss of respiratory muscle tone, allowing the abdominal contents to push the diaphragm cranially. Other groups have, however, found only minor displacement of the diaphragm with the anterior part even being shifted caudally.[4] Such

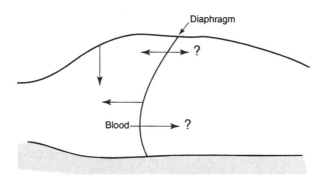

Fig 9.1   Changes in chest wall configuration during anaesthesia. There is a slight decrease in the transverse chest area. The top of the diaphragm dome is moved cranially. Some studies suggest a caudal displacement of the anterior part of the diaphragm whereas others do not. There is also some controversy regarding blood volume shifts. Studies with measurement of pulmonary blood volume (or central blood volume) by indicator dilution technique suggest a decreased intrathoracic blood volume during anaesthesia and mechanical ventilation.

caudal displacement could in theory occur if the ribs are tilted downwards during anaesthesia.

Airway closure

It has been shown in awake, healthy, human volunteers that airways in dependent lung regions close during a deep expiration, as discussed in chapter 5. Gas can be trapped in the lungs during anaesthesia and can be released by deep inflations. This suggests that airway closure occurs during ordinary breathing in the anaesthetised patient.[3] It has also been shown that a decrease of FRC during anaesthesia below the awake closing capacity (CC—the lung volume at which airways close) was accompanied by a significantly larger shunt (mean 11%) than when FRC during anaesthesia was larger than the awake CC (mean 2%).[5] The importance of airway closure in the anaesthetised patient is, however, still under debate. Additional and perhaps more important functional disturbances may impede arterial oxygenation, as seen below.

Atelectasis

In a classic paper by Bendixen and co-workers, a decreasing compliance and Pao_2 were seen during anaesthesia. The authors suggested that these changes were an effect of increasing formation of atelectasis.[6] Other research groups, however, found an immediate decrease in lung compliance on induction of anaesthesia with no further deterioration during the anaesthesia period. Moreover, it has not been possible to demonstrate regular occurrence of atelectasis by means of conventional radiographs. This turned opinion away from atelectasis as the cause of altered lung mechanics and impaired gas exchange during anaesthesia. In the mid-1980s, however, new observations were made that may explain the altered mechanical behaviour of the lung during anaesthesia. Using computed tomography with transverse exposures, prompt development of densities in dependent regions of both lungs could be demonstrated in the anaesthetised patient (Fig 9.2). Similar densities had been seen previously in anaesthetised infants.[7] Morphological studies in various animals proved the same kind of densities to be atelectasis. The atelectasis appears in almost 90% of all patients anaesthetised; it is independent of age and is only loosely related to body configuration. The atelectasis appears during spontaneous breathing and after muscle paralysis, whether anaesthesia is inhalational or intravenous.

Spiral computed tomography enables a complete description of changes in lung aeration, as well as the formation of atelectasis, during general anaesthesia. By using this technique, it was shown that the formation of atelectasis occurs in a gravitationally oriented fashion (that is, in dependent lung regions), but also with a non-gravitational inhomogeneity (increasing

(a)

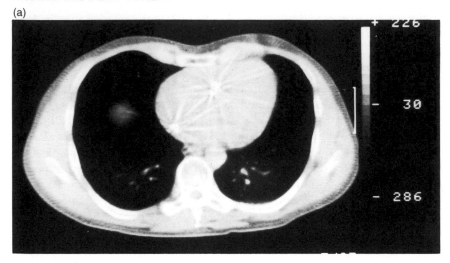

(b)

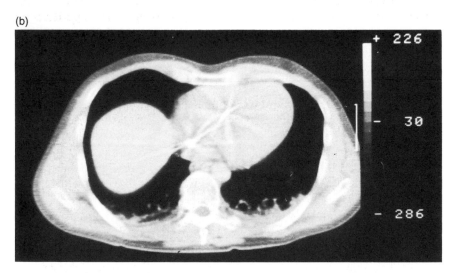

Fig 9.2 Computed tomography with transverse exposures of the chest when the subject is (a) awake and then (b) anaesthetised. Note the well aerated lung in the awake condition. A few pulmonary vessels can be seen in the lower lung regions. The radiating beams in the heart are caused by a catheter that is positioned with its tip in the pulmonary artery. During anaesthesia, atelectasis has developed in the most dependent regions of both lungs (seen as grey/white irregular areas). The large grey/white area in the middle of the right lung field is caused by a cranial shift of the diaphragm and the underlying liver. The exposure levels of the two scans are the same relative to the spine.

atelectasis from apex to base) (Fig 9.3).[7] The effect on gas exchange is dealt with later.

Prevention of atelectasis

As atelectasis is recurrent during anaesthesia (and causes shunt and impaired oxygenation of the blood, as discussed later) its prevention, or the reopening of already collapsed lung tissue, should be of interest. Different methods that have been applied are discussed below: (1) positive end expiratory pressure (PEEP); (2) maintenance or restoration of respiratory muscle tone; (3) recruitment manoeuvres; and (4) minimisation of pulmonary gas resorption.

Positive end expiratory pressure

The application of PEEP has been tested in several studies and will consistently re-open collapsed lung tissue.[7] PEEP appears, however, not to be the ideal procedure. First, shunt is not reduced and the arterial oxygenation is not improved on average in larger groups—some patients get better but others may get worse. The maintenance of shunt may be explained by the redistribution of blood flow towards the most dependent

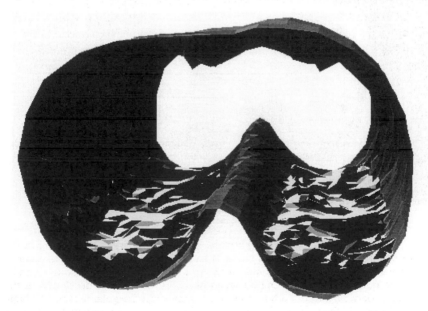

Fig 9.3 A three dimensional reconstruction of the thorax of an anaesthetised patient with atelectasis in the dependent regions of both lungs. Note the irregular shape of the atelectasis. There is a slight decrease in the amount of atelectasis towards the apex which is at the distal end of the chest wall on the image. (Reproduced by courtesy of Dr A Reber.)

parts when intrathoracic pressure is increased, so that any persisting atelectasis in the bottom of the lung receives a larger share of the pulmonary blood flow than without PEEP.[8] The increased intrathoracic pressure will also impede venous return and lower cardiac output. This results in a lower venous O_2 tension for a given O_2 uptake, which will augment the desaturating effect of shunted blood and perfusion of poorly ventilated regions on the arterial oxygenation. Second, the lung re-collapses rapidly after discontinuation of PEEP. Within one minute of this cessation of PEEP, the collapse is as large as it was before its application. This means that, to bring the patient through the intraoperative period without lung collapse, the PEEP must be maintained without interruption; this must also happen during the wake up and early postoperative periods.

Maintenance of muscle tone

The use of an anaesthetic that allows maintenance of respiratory muscle tone prevents atelectasis formation. Ketamine maintains tone and is the only anaesthetic so far studied that does not cause atelectasis if administered alone. If a muscle relaxant is given together with ketamine, however, atelectasis will appear as with other anaesthetics.[7]

Another attempt is to restore respiratory muscle function which can be achieved, at least partly, by diaphragm pacing. This has been tested by applying phrenic nerve stimulation, which reduced the atelectatic area.[7] The effect was, however, small and it can be argued that the technique is too complicated to become routine during anaesthesia and surgery.

Recruitment manoeuvres

The use of a sigh manoeuvre, or a double tidal volume, has frequently been advocated to re-open any collapsed lung tissue. The atelectasis is not, however, affected by an ordinary tidal volume, to an end inspiratory airway pressure of 10 cm H_2O, or by a deep sigh with an airway pressure to $+20$ cm H_2O.[1] Not until an airway pressure of 30 cm H_2O is reached does the atelectasis decrease to about half the initial value. For a complete re-opening of all collapsed lung tissue, an inflation pressure of 40 cm H_2O is required, and the breath must be held for 15 s. Such a large inflation, and subsequent expiration down to -20 cm H_2O, corresponds to a vital capacity measured during spontaneous breathing with the patient awake. Such a manoeuvre may be considered risky and cause baro-/volotrauma. Another procedure has therefore been tested with repeated inflations of the lung to an airway pressure of $+30$ cm H_2O. This, however, causes only a small degree of further opening of the lung tissue after the first manoeuvre. A full vital capacity manoeuvre with an inflation to $+40$ cm H_2O therefore seems necessary to completely re-open the lung.

Table 9.1   Procedures to prevent atelectasis during anaesthesia

Procedure	Effects
Apply PEEP	Reduced cardiac output, no improvement in Pa_{O_2}, no effect after discontinuation
Maintain respiratory muscle tone, that is, ketamine anaesthesia	Interference with surgery?
Stimulate phrenic nerve, that is, diaphragm pacing	Small effect?
Perform a "vital capacity manoeuvre" ($Paw = 40$ cm H_2O)	Baro/volotrauma?
Avoid high oxygen fraction during anaesthesia	Hypoxaemia?
Avoid 100% O_2 during induction of anaesthesia	Hypoxaemia?

Minimising gas resorption

Ventilation of the lungs with pure O_2, after a vital capacity manoeuvre that had re-opened previously collapsed lung tissue, results in a rapid reappearance of atelectasis. If, on the other hand, ventilation is made with 40% O_2 in N_2, atelectasis reappears slowly and is still minor 30–40 minutes after the inflation manoeuvre. Thus, ventilation during anaesthesia should be done with a moderate inspired O_2 fraction (for example, 0·3–0·4) and be increased only if arterial oxygenation is compromised. Moreover, avoidance of the preoxygenation procedure during induction of anaesthesia more or less eliminates the atelectasis formation during anaesthesia.[9] Thus, avoidance of preoxygenation or, possibly, lowering of inspired O_2 fraction during the induction phase reduces or avoids the formation of atelectasis during subsequent anaesthesia. It is obvious that lowering of the inspired O_2 fraction may increase the risk of hypoxaemia in a difficult and prolonged intubation of the airway. It may, however, be that induction of anaesthesia with an inspired O_2 fraction of 50–80% is enough to ensure safe oxygenation. Moreover, the obligatory use of pulse oximeters during anaesthesia in many countries makes it easy to detect dangerous hypoxaemia. Moderate oxygen concentrations during induction of anaesthesia, and intermittent "vital capacity" manoeuvres during the anaesthesia and surgery, may well be worth a larger trial!

The different procedures for preventing atelectasis formation, or re-opening collapsed lung tissue, are listed in Table 9.1.

1 Don H. The mechanical properties of the respiratory system during anesthesia. *Int Anesthesiol Clin* 1977;**15**:113–36.
2 Rehder K, Sessler AD, Marsh HM. General anesthesia and the lung. In: Murray JF, ed. *Lung disease: state of the art*. New York: American Lung Association, 1975–1976: 367–89.
3 Wahba RWM. Perioperative functional residual capacity. *Can J Anaesth* 1991;**38**:384–400.
4 Rehder K, Hedenstierna G. Lung function during anesthesia: solved and unresolved questions: Anniversary editorial. *Curr Opin Anesthesiol* 1997;**10**:viii–xi.
5 Dueck R, Prutow RJ, Davies NJ, Clausen JL, Davidson TM. The lung volume at which

shunting occurs with inhalation anesthesia. *Anesthesiology* 1988;**69**:854–61.

6 Bendixen HH, Hedley-Whyte J, Laver MB. Impaired oxygenation in surgical patients during general anesthesia with controlled ventilation: a concept of atelectasis. *N Engl J Med* 1963;**269**:991–6.

7 Hedenstierna G. Ventilation–perfusion relationships during anaesthesia. *Thorax* 1995;**50**:85–91.

8 West JB, Dollery CT, Naimark A. Distribution of blood flow in isolated lung: relation to vascular and alveolar pressures. *J Appl Physiol* 1964;**19**:713–24.

9 Rothen HU, Sporre B, Engberg G, Wegenius G, Reber A, Hedenstierna G. Prevention of atelectasis during general anaesthesia. *Lancet* 1995;**345**:1387–91.

10: Ventilation, blood flow, and gas exchange during anaesthesia

Distribution of ventilation

Wash out studies using multiple breath nitrogen in anaesthetised, supine humans during spontaneous breathing and mechanical ventilation have shown no clear change in the overall ventilation distribution index (that is, gas mixing efficiency) compared with the awake state. More interesting data have been obtained when studying gas distribution in each lung separately in the lateral position during anaesthesia, by means of a double lumen endobronchial catheter. These studies indicate a larger ventilation of the upper lung than has been seen in awake, spontaneously breathing patients.[1] Using isotope techniques, a similar redistribution of inspired gas from dependent to non-dependent lung regions has been observed in anaesthetised supine humans. Thus, using a radiolabelled aerosol and single photon emission computed tomography (SPECT), ventilation was shown to be distributed mainly to the upper lung regions, and there was a successive decrease down the lower half of the lung.[2] Moreover, there was no ventilation at all in the bottom of the lung, corresponding to the distribution of atelectasis that was simultaneously obtained by computed tomography (Fig 10.1).

Positive end expiratory pressure (PEEP) increases dependent lung ventilation in anaesthetised patients in the lateral position, so that ventilation distribution is more similar to that in the awake state. Similar findings of more even distribution between upper and lower lung regions have also been made in supine, anaesthetised humans after a previous inflation of the lungs, similar to PEEP.[3] Thus, restoration of overall functional residual capacity (FRC) towards, or beyond, the awake level returns gas distribution towards the awake pattern. It is tempting to attribute this to recruitment of collapsed, dependent lung regions (atelectasis) and re-opening of closed airways in lower lung regions, and possibly to increased expansion of upper lung regions, so that these become less compliant.

Distribution of lung blood flow

The distribution of lung blood flow has recently been studied by the injection of radioactively labelled macroaggregated albumin and SPECT in anaesthetised, mechanically ventilated patients.[2] A successive increase of perfusion down the lung, from ventral to dorsal aspects, was seen, with some reduction in the lowermost region. Thus, the lowermost portion of the lung, which was atelectatic as evidenced by simultaneous computed tomography, was still perfused (Fig 10.1).

Positive end expiratory pressure will impede the venous return to the right heart and therefore reduce cardiac output. It may also affect pulmonary vascular resistance, although this may have less effect on cardiac output. In addition, PEEP causes a redistribution of blood flow towards dependent lung regions.[4] By this means upper lung regions may be poorly perfused, causing an effect similar to dead space. Moreover, forcing of the blood volume down to the dorsal side of the lungs, if the patient is supine, may increase the fractional blood flow through an atelectatic region.[5]

Several inhalational anaesthetics have been found to inhibit the hypoxic pulmonary vasoconstriction (HPV) in isolated lung preparations. No such effect has, however, been seen with intravenous anaesthetics (barbiturates).[6] Results from human studies vary, and can be explained reasonably

(a)

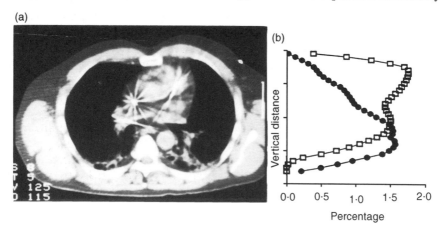

(b)

Vertical distance

0·0   0·5   1·0   1·5   2·0

Percentage

Fig 10.1   (a) Transverse CT scan with atelectasis visible in the dependent parts of both lungs and (b) corresponding vertical distributions of ventilation and lung blood flow in an anaesthetised subject. Note that ventilation (□) is distributed preferentially to upper lung regions, contrary to what is seen in an awake subject. Note also the decreasing ventilation in the lower part and the complete cessation of ventilation in the bottom, corresponding to the atelectatic area. Perfusion (●), on the other hand, increases down the lung, except for the bottommost region where a decrease can be seen. This so called zone IV may be caused by increased interstitial lung pressure compressing extra-alveolar vessels, and hypoxic pulmonary vasoconstriction.

by the complexity of the experiment, which causes several variables to change at the same time. The HPV response may thus be obscured by simultaneous changes in cardiac output, myocardial contractility, vascular tone, blood volume distribution, blood pH and CO_2 tension, and lung mechanics. In studies with no gross changes in cardiac output, the inhalational anaesthetics isoflurane and halothane depress the HPV response by 50% at 2 MAC (minimum alveolar concentration).[6]

Dead space, shunt, and ventilation–perfusion relationships

Both CO_2 elimination and oxygenation of blood are impaired in most patients during anaesthesia. The impeded CO_2 elimination can be attributed to an increased dead space ventilation. Single breath, washout recordings have demonstrated that "anatomical" dead space is unchanged, indicating that the "alveolar" or parallel dead space must have been increased during anaesthesia.[7] Using a sophisticated multiple inert gas elimination technique (described in Part III), it can be shown that the increased CO_2 dead space during anaesthesia is not really a dead space but poorly perfused lung regions, which are signified by so called "high $\dot{V}A/\dot{Q}$" ratios. Such "high $\dot{V}A/\dot{Q}$" ratios can be explained by the tiny perfusion of corner vessels in interalveolar septa in the upper lung regions (where alveolar pressure may exceed pulmonary vascular pressure—zone I).[8] The impaired CO_2 elimination is on the whole easily accounted for by increasing the ventilation and is seldom a problem in routine anaesthesia with mechanical ventilation.

The impairment of arterial oxygenation during anaesthesia is generally considered to be more severe at higher ages; obesity worsens the oxygenation of blood and smokers show more gas exchange impairment than non-smokers.[9] Venous admixture, as calculated according to the standard O_2 "shunt" equation, is also increased during anaesthesia to about 10% of cardiac output. The venous admixture, however, includes not only perfusion of non-ventilated lung tissue (true shunt), but also regions that are poorly ventilated or perfused in excess of their ventilation ("low $\dot{V}A/\dot{Q}$ regions"). The multiple inert gas elimination technique (discussed later) enables the construction of a virtually continuous distribution of ventilation–perfusion ratios. In young healthy volunteers studied by this technique during anaesthesia, with thiopentone and methoxyflurane, both ventilation and perfusion were distributed to wider ranges of $\dot{V}A/\dot{Q}$ ratios, which can be expressed as an increase in the logarithmic standard deviation of the perfusion distribution (log $SD\dot{Q}$). In a similar group of patients studied during halothane anaesthesia and muscle paralysis, log $SD\dot{Q}$ was almost doubled, from 0·43 when awake to 0·80 during anaesthesia. In addition, true shunt was increased to a mean of 8%. A similar increase in shunt from

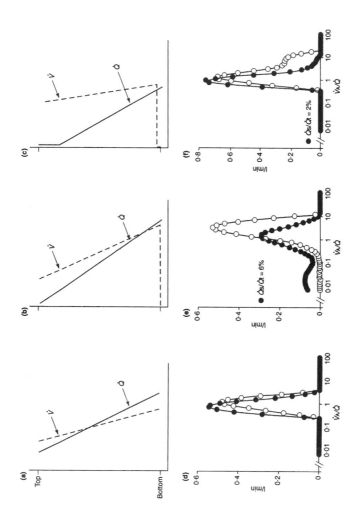

Fig 10.2 Schematic drawings of the vertical distributions of ventilation and blood flow (upper panels) and corresponding $\dot{V}A/\dot{Q}$ distributions (lower panels) in a subject (a) when awake, and during anaesthesia (b) without end expiratory pressure (ZEEP) and (c) with a positive end expiratory pressure of 10 cm H_2O (PEEP). The recordings during the awake state are the same as those shown in Fig 8.1. Note the considerable change in the ventilation distribution during anaesthesia and the similarity with the isotope measurements in Fig 10.1. Corresponding $\dot{V}A/\dot{Q}$ distribution (d, e, f) shows shunt and regions with low $\dot{V}A/\dot{Q}$ ratios. In addition, there is more ventilation to high $\dot{V}A/\dot{Q}$ (○) regions than in the awake state. With the application of PEEP perfusion (●) of low $\dot{V}A/\dot{Q}$ regions is abolished and shunt is reduced. There is, however, more ventilation to high $\dot{V}A/\dot{Q}$ regions.

Table 10.1 Ventilation–perfusion relationships during anaesthesia

	$\dot{Q}$mean	log SD$\dot{Q}$	$\dot{V}$mean	log SD$\dot{V}$	Shunt (%$\dot{Q}_T$)	Dead space (%V_T)	Pa_{O_2}/F_{IO_2} (kPa)
Awake	0·76 (0·33)	0·68 (0·28)	1·11 (0·52)	0·52 (0·15)	0·5 (1·0)	34·8 (14·2)	59·5 (8·1)
Anaesthetised	0·65 (0·34)	1·04 (0·36)	1·38 (0·76)	0·76 (0·31)	4·8 (4·1)	35·0 (9·9)	50·9 (15·2)

Mean (SD) ventilation–perfusion relationships with no cardiopulmonary disease (normal, $n=45$), awake and during general anaesthesia and muscle paralysis. F_{IO_2} (inspired oxygen fraction) awake: 0·21; anaesthetised: 0·42.

1% awake to a mean of 9% during anaesthesia was recorded in a study on middle aged (37–64 years) surgical patients, and there was a widening of the $\dot{V}_A/\dot{Q}$ distribution (log SD$\dot{Q}$=0·47 when awake, 1·01 during anaesthesia).[4] A schematic example of a $\dot{V}_A/\dot{Q}$ distribution is given in Fig 10.2. In elderly patients with more severe impairment of lung function, halothane anaesthesia with muscle paralysis, with or without nitrous oxide, caused considerable widening of the $\dot{V}_A/\dot{Q}$ distribution with log SD$\dot{Q}$ increasing from 0·87 when awake to 1·73 during anaesthesia. In addition, shunt increased to a mean of 15%, with a large variation between patients (0–30%).[4] Thus, the most consistent findings during anaesthesia are an increased $\dot{V}_A/\dot{Q}$ mismatch, expressed as an increased log SD$\dot{Q}$, and an increase in shunt.

More recently, the $\dot{V}_A/\dot{Q}$ distribution has been correlated with CT findings during anaesthesia. The major $\dot{V}_A/\dot{Q}$ disturbance was once again shunt and very little of low $\dot{V}_A/\dot{Q}$ ratio.[4] A good correlation between the magnitude of shunt and the size of atelectasis was seen. PEEP can reduce

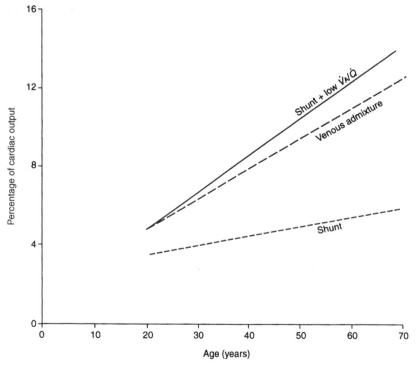

Fig 10.3 The influence of age on shunt, shunt + low $\dot{V}_A/\dot{Q}$, and venous admixture in anaesthetised patients. There is a slight and insignificant increase in shunt with age whereas shunt + low $\dot{V}_A/\dot{Q}$ increases rapidly. Note also that venous admixture is more similar to shunt + perfusion of low $\dot{V}_A/\dot{Q}$ regions than to shunt alone. (From Gunnarsson et al.[10]).

the atelectatic area but the effect on shunt varies; in some patients it falls and in others it increases. As mentioned earlier, the continuing shunt despite PEEP can probably be explained by a redistribution of blood flow towards dependent, still atelectatic regions.[5] The intravenous anaesthetic agent ketamine, which does not produce any atelectasis, does not cause any shunt as assessed by the multiple inert gas elimination technique, whereas both can be seen when the patient is paralysed with a muscle relaxant. Atelectasis and shunt do not increase with the age of the patient when data from several studies are pooled.[10] On the other hand, perfusion of regions with low $\dot{V}A/\dot{Q}$ ratios increases with both anaesthesia and age (Fig 10.3). One probable explanation for the increased mismatch (increased log $SD\dot{Q}$) is the previously discussed airway closure, which is known to become more important with age in the awake subject.[11] Normal values for more important variables that can be derived from the multiple inert gas data are shown in Table 10.1.

1 Rehder K, Hatch DJ, Sessler AD, Fowler WS. The function of each lung of anesthetized and paralyzed man during mechanical ventilation. *Anesthesiology* 1972;**37**:16–26.
2 Tokics L, Hedenstierna G, Svensson L, Brismar B, Cederlund T, Lundquist H, Strandberg A. *V/Q* distribution and correlation to atelectasis in anesthetized paralyzed humans. *J Appl Physiol* 1996;**1**:1822–33.
3 Hulands GH, Greene R, Iliff LD, Nunn JF. Influence of anaesthesia on the regional distribution of perfusion and ventilation in the lung. *Clin Sci* 1970;**38**:451–60.
4 Hedenstierna G. Ventilation–perfusion relationships during anaesthesia. *Thorax* 1995;**50**:85–91.
5 Bendixen HH, Hedley-Whyte J, Laver MB. Impaired oxygenation in surgical patients during general anesthesia with controlled ventilation: a concept of atelectasis. *N Engl J Med* 1963;**269**:991–6.
6 Marshall BE. Effects of anesthetics on pulmonary gas exchange. In: Stanley TH, Sperry RJ, eds. *Anesthesia and the lung*. London: Kluwer Academic, 1989: 117–25.
7 Nunn JF, Hill DW. Respiratory dead space and arterial to endtidal CO_2 tension difference in anaesthetized man. *J Appl Physiol* 1960;**15**:383–9.
8 Hedenstierna G, White FC, Mazzone R, Wagner PD. Redistribution of pulmonary blood flow in the dog with positive end-expiratory pressure ventilation. *J Appl Physiol* 1979;**46**:278–87.
9 Nunn JF. *Nunn's applied respiratory physiology*, 4th edn. Oxford: Heinemann 1993: 407–8.
10 Gunnarsson L, Tokics L, Gustavsson, Hedenstierna G. Influence of age on atelectasis formation and gas exchange impairment during general anaesthesia. *Br J Anaesth* 1991;**66**:423–32.
11 Leblanc P, Ruff F, Milic Emili J. Effects of age and body position on "airway closure" in man. *J Appl Physiol* 1970;**28**:448–51.

11: Pulmonary densities and respiratory mechanics in ARDS

Acute respiratory distress syndrome (ARDS) is characterised by pulmonary infiltrates,[1] which were earlier considered to be rather homogeneously distributed over the lung. Thus, conventional chest radiographs showed densities in both dependent and independent regions, the so called "snow storm" lung (Fig 11.1a). The infiltrates are caused by extravasation of fluid, producing protein rich pulmonary oedema, which is followed by fibrosis. These changes are accompanied by a functional disturbance, the hallmarks of which are hypoxaemia and stiffness of the lung (reduced compliance). Recently, more or less established concepts have been challenged, calling for a review of the present knowledge of the distribution of morphology and pathophysiology of the ARDS lung.

Pulmonary densities

In the mid-1980s, new aspects on the distribution of lung pathology in ARDS were presented. They were the result of the application of computed tomography (CT) in the intensive care setting. These papers challenged the commonly held opinion that ARDS is a generalised disease.[2] The authors found patchy infiltrates, interspersed with areas of normal appearing lung, in transverse exposures of the chest. Moreover, most of the densities were found in the dependent regions, indicating an influence of gravitational forces (Fig 11.1b). The densities had an attenuation of around 0 hounsfield units (HU), indicating airlessness. They were thus qualitatively similar to the densities (atelectasis) seen during anaesthesia, but quantitatively much larger. Thus, in ARDS patients densities may account for up to 70–80% of the lungfield, compared with 4–8% in the lungs of healthy, anaesthetised patients. The apical regions appeared to be less compromised whereas the hilar and basal regions were more affected. When the patient was turned from the supine to the prone position, the densities moved from the paravertebral to the sternal regions. Thus, the densities moved within minutes, from the previously dependent to the newly dependent regions of the lung. The rapid redistribution can hardly be explained by formation of new oedema in dependent regions and reabsorption of earlier oedema in non-dependent lung levels—reabsorption takes hours and even days.[3] The changes in the CT densities are also too great to be explained by a blood volume shift. The most likely explanation is redistribution of intra-pulmonary gas, caused by compression of dependent lung regions by the increased weight of the lung.

Surprisingly, the vertical fractional distribution of the tissue mass in the ARDS lung is similar to that in normal subjects. Thus, the regional tissue mass is more than twice the normal mass all over the lung.[4] This suggests that oedema does not accumulate in dependent lung regions only but is distributed evenly over the lungfield. As alveoli are, however, less distended

(a)

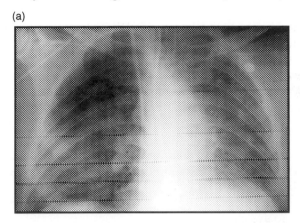

(b)

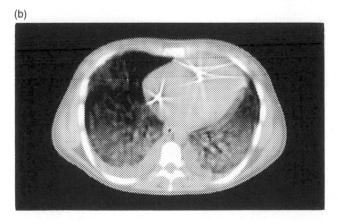

Fig 11.1 (a) Frontal chest radiograph and (b) corresponding transverse CT scan in a patient with ARDS. Note the rather homogeneous distribution of densities in the conventional chest radiograph and the gravitational distribution of the densities on the CT scan. (By courtesy of Dr Pelosi, Milan, Italy.)

in dependent regions than in upper, non-dependent regions (see chapter 5), the amount of tissue per unit of volume increases down the lung. Thus, most of the oedema is located in the dependent regions of the lung, giving the visual impression of non-homogeneous, gravitational distribution of lung damage.

With increasing positive end expiratory pressure (PEEP), substantial clearing of lung regions of high density is the recurrent finding. The amount of normally inflated lung tissue increases significantly whereas the non-inflated tissue decreases, indicating alveolar recruitment. Also, the application of, or increase in, PEEP reduces the shunt (as it reduces the amount of non-aerated tissues).[2]

The attenuation numbers of the CT scan can be used to calculate the weight of the lung. It averaged 2·6 kg in a group of patients with severe ARDS, which is close to the lung weight found *post mortem* in patients with ARDS (mean 2·5 kg).[5] This is also twice the weight found in normal subjects studied by computed tomography.[5] Despite collapse of alveoli in the ARDS lung, the dimension of the lung is not reduced, as evidenced by the maintained transverse area of the lung on the CT scan. This suggests that gas volume has been replaced by an equal amount of fluid (although a shift of the position of the diaphragm may influence the total lung volume).

The increased leakage of the pulmonary vessels that has been assumed for a long time has more recently been demonstrated by gamma camera technique and positron emission tomography (PET).[6] These studies show that the capillary leakage is increased almost tenfold during the first days of ARDS and remains elevated at about five times the normal a week or more later. Moreover, the capillary leakage was elevated even when the extravascular density had been reduced or had approached normal, which may suggest an increased drainage of the pulmonary tissue.

Respiratory mechanics

One of the hallmarks of ARDS is the reduction of lung compliance. The ARDS lung is usually referred to as a "stiff lung" as a result of the high pressures needed to inflate it. When ARDS patients were studied using computed tomography and recording of the static volume–pressure curve of the lung, it was found that lung compliance was significantly correlated with the amount of normally inflated lung.[7] On the other hand, there was no correlation between lung compliance and the amount of poorly inflated or non-inflated, collapsed tissue. The findings suggest that compliance is correlated to the air containing part of the lung and not to the "amount of disease" (although oedema accumulation expels air out of the lung, as mentioned above). These findings have been given the nickname "baby lung" in ARDS.

Over the past few years it has been shown that inspiratory resistance in the anaesthetised and mechanically ventilated patient is much higher than previously believed, and that the tissue component is more important than the airway component, that is, resistive forces in the tissue exert greater impedance to the inspiration than the resistance to airflow in the airways.[8] Moreover, established facts have also been challenged by showing that resistance increases with lung volume and decreases with airflow, contrary to previous concepts.[8] Again, the volume and flow dependence are the result of the dominating tissue resistance. The tissue resistance is also clearly increased in ARDS.[9] What causes the tissue resistance to increase in ARDS is not clear. It seems to occur early during ARDS, and may therefore reflect oedema rather than fibrosis.

1 Ashbaugh DG, Bigelow DB, Petty TL, Levine BE. Acute respiratory distress in adults. *Lancet* 1967;**ii**:319–23.
2 Rommelsheim K, Lakner K, Westhofen P, Distelmaier W, Hirt S. Das respiratorische Distress-Syndrome der Erwachsenen (ARDS) im Computer Tomogram. *Anasth Intensivther Notfallmed* 1983;**18**:59–64.
3 Staub NC. New concepts about the pathophysiology of pulmonary edema. *J Thorac Imaging* 1988;**3**:8–14.
4 Gattinoni L, Pelosi P, Vitale G, Pesenti A, D'Andrea L, Mascheroni D. Body position changes redistribute lung computed-tomographic density in patients with acute respiratory failure. *Anesthesiology* 1991;**74**:15–23.
5 Gattinoni L, Pesenti A, Bombino M, Baglioni S, Rivolta M, Rossi F, et al. Relationships between lung computed tomographic density, gas exchange, and PEEP in acute respiratory failure. *Anesthesiology* 1988;**69**:824–32.
6 Calandrino FS Jr, Anderson DJ, Mintun MA, Schuster DP. Pulmonary vascular permeability during the adult respiratory distress syndrome: a positron emission tomographic study. *Am Rev Respir Dis* 1988;**138**:421–8.
7 Gattinoni L, Pesenti A, Avalli L, Rossi F, Bombino M. Pressure–volume curve of total respiratory system in acute respiratory failure. Computed tomographic scan study. *Am Rev Respir Dis* 1987;**136**:730–6.
8 Gottfried SB, Rossi A, Higgs BD, Calverley PM, Zocchi L, Bozic C, Milic-Emili J. Noninvasive determination of respiratory system mechanics during mechanical ventilation for acute respiratory failure. *Am Rev Respir Dis* 1985;**131**:414–20.
9 Tantucci C, Corbeil C, Chasse M, Braidy J, Matar N, Milic-Emili J. Flow resistance in patients with chronic obstructive pulmonary disease in acute respiratory failure. Effects of flow and volume. *Am Rev Respir Dis* 1991;**144**:384–9.

12: Ventilation, circulation, and gas exchange in ARDS

Ventilation distribution

The ventilation distribution has been assessed in patients with acute respiratory distress syndrome (ARDS) by comparing computed tomography (CT) scans taken at end inspiration and end expiration.[1] Ventilation went preferentially to upper lung regions at no or low levels of positive end expiratory pressure (PEEP), a finding that may not be too surprising in view of the collapse or consolidation of dependent lung regions, which has been shown so nicely in a large number of studies by this group. With increasing PEEP, the distribution of ventilation became more and more homogeneous,[1] that is, ventilation of dependent regions increased. When it comes to the oxygenation of blood and elimination of CO_2, the distribution of ventilation should match that of blood flow. As described previously (see chapter 5), perfusion of the healthy lung is mainly distributed to dependent parts. Even in severe ARDS, it can be anticipated that there is a persisting blood flow through the lower lung units, producing the shunt. In other words, it must be advantageous, in terms of gas exchange, to increase ventilation of dependent regions. A large inspiration seems to cause damage to the lung. This is called volo-/barotrauma.[2] Thus, attempts to improve ventilation of dependent lung regions by the application of PEEP may, in theory, cause damage to upper lung regions. This is because of the larger initial inflation of the upper lung regions. In ARDS, however, the damage seems to predominate in the lower lung regions.[3] This has been proposed as being the result of "shear stress failure", that is, the opening and closing of lung units with each tidal breath.[4] If this is the mechanism, PEEP should be advocated to prevent intermittent collapse of lung units. It is thus like sailing between Scylla and Charybd—too much PEEP may cause volotrauma and too little promote shear stress failure. A formula that has been proposed is to apply high enough PEEP to prevent shear stress failure *and* low tidal volume to prevent volotrauma, thus allowing the arterial P_{CO_2} to increase—so called "permissive hypercapnia".[5]

Pulmonary circulation

A frequent finding in ARDS is pulmonary hypertension.[6] When comparing pulmonary artery pressure and data from CT scans, a good correlation between mean pulmonary artery pressure and lung weight has been shown.[7] It is not clear what is the cause and what the effect. An increase in pulmonary artery pressure may induce an increase of lung oedema, that is, an increase in lung weight. On the other hand, an oedematous lung may lead to an increase in pulmonary artery pressure by compression of pulmonary vessels. Whichever the independent variable, an average of 133 Pa (1 mm Hg) increase of pulmonary artery pressure was associated with a 14% increase in lung weight.[7]

Gas exchange

Although lung compliance is correlated with the normally inflated part of the lung (see above), the gas exchange impairment is strongly related to the amount of disease, that is, the non-inflated tissue mass. Thus, the impairment of arterial oxygenation and the venous admixture ("shunt") correlate with the quantity of non-inflated lung tissue.[7] This suggests that the shunt fraction (that is, perfusion of the non-inflated tissue) is the main cause of hypoxaemia in patients with ARDS. It is likely, however, that the non-inflated tissue is relatively underperfused as evidenced by the discrepancy between the shunt fraction and the non-inflated tissue fraction (for example, 30% of shunt with 60% of non-inflated tissue). This may indicate some effects of mechanical compression of vessels in the consolidated region, and persisting hypoxic pulmonary vasoconstriction. This has been shown in experimental oleic acid oedema—dependent, consolidated lung regions being less perfused than during baseline, before oedema[8] (Fig 12.1).

The correlation between the amount of non-aerated lung tissue and hypoxaemia and venous admixture might be anticipated. Venous admixture does not, however, separate true shunt (perfusion of non-ventilated, atelectatic, or consolidated lung regions) from regions that are poorly ventilated in relation to their blood flow (low $\dot{V}_A/\dot{Q}$). In studies on ARDS patients with the multiple inert gas elimination technique for assessing the distribution of $\dot{V}_A/\dot{Q}$ ratios, the major finding has been a large shunt, from 20% to 70% of cardiac output.[9] Some patients may, in addition, show increased perfusion of low $\dot{V}_A/\dot{Q}$ regions but most have few other disturbances. This fits with non-aerated tissue being the major or single cause of hypoxaemia in ARDS, by producing shunt regions. Thus, the alveoli demonstrate quantal behaviour, being either ventilated and perfused, or not ventilated at all but perfused (the possibility remains that there are also alveoli that are neither ventilated nor perfused—they will not show

73

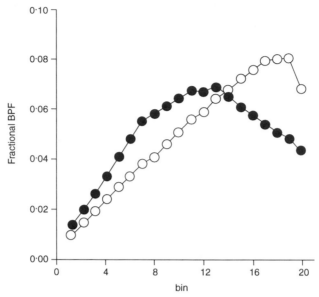

Fig 12.1   The vertical perfusion of the lung of a dog (o) before and after (•) oleic acid oedema. Note the persisting (although slightly reduced) blood flow in the dependent lung regions after creation of lung oedema induced by oleic acid. The dependent regions are where atelectasis and consolidation can be expected (compare Fig 11.1). (From Schuster,[8] with permission of the author and the publisher.)

up on the $\dot{V}A/\dot{Q}$ distribution obtained by the multiple inert gas elimination technique).

1 Gattinoni L, Pelosi P, Crotti S, Valenza F. Effects of positive end-expiratory pressure on regional distribution of tidal volume and recruitment in adult respiratory distress syndrome. *Am J Respir Crit Care Med* 1995;**151**:1807–14.
2 Dreyfuss D, Saumon G. Role of tidal volume, FRC, and end-inspiratory volume in the development of pulmonary edema following mechanical ventilation. Am Rev Respir Dis 1993;**148**:1194–203.
3 Gattinoni L, Bombino M, Pelosi P, Lissoni A, Pesenti A, Fumagalli R, Tagliabue M. Lung structure and function in different stages of severe adult respiratory distress syndrome. *JAMA* 1994;**271**:1772–9.
4 Muscedere JG, Mullen JB, Gan K, Slutsky AS. Tidal ventilation at low airway pressures can augment lung injury. *Am J Respir Crit Care Med* 1994;**149**:1327–34.
5 Amato MB, Barbas CS, Medeiros DM, Schettino G de P, Lorenzi-Filho G, Kairalla RA, et al. Beneficial effects of the "open lung approach" with low distending pressures in acute respiratory distress syndrome. A prospective randomized study on mechanical ventilation. *Am J Respir Crit Care Med* 1995;**152**:1835–46.
6 Ashbaugh DG, Bigelow DB, Petty TL, Levine BE. Acute respiratory distress in adults. *Lancet* 1967;**ii**:319–23.
7 Gattinoni L, Pesenti A, Bombino M, Baglioni S, Rivolta M, Rossi F, et al. Relationships between lung computed tomographic density, gas exchange, and PEEP in acute respiratory failure. *Anesthesiology* 1988;**69**:824–32.

8 Schuster DP. ARDS: Clinical lessons from this oleic acid model of acute lung injury. State of the art. *Am J Respir Crit Care Med* 1994;**149**:245–60.

9 Ashbaugh DG, Petty TL, Bigelow DB, Harris TM. Continuous positive-pressure breathing (CPPB) in adult respiratory distress syndrome. *J Thorac Cardiovasc Surg* 1969;**57**:31–41.

Part III

Practice of respiratory measurement

This part deals with the assessment of respiratory function, with emphasis on measurements in the anaesthetised patient, both during spontaneous breathing and during mechanical ventilation. As will be seen, there are large differences between the two, in what can be measured, how to do the measurement, and how to interpret the results. Measurements of the following are discussed: (1) ventilation, where differences in applicable techniques between the two states are small; (2) lung volumes; (3) gas distribution; (4) respiratory mechanics, where large differences exist in what can be studied and how to do it awake and anaesthetised subjects; and (5) gas exchange, including diffusion and ventilation–perfusion ($\dot{V}A/\dot{Q}$) matching.

13:   Measurement of ventilation

Measurement of ventilation may appear to be a simple task, but it has emerged as more complicated than most realise. This is because temperature, humidity, pressure, viscosity, and density all affect the recording of gas volume, and thus of ventilation (volume per unit time). In addition, leaks in the recording and collecting systems of respiratory gas cause losses of or false increases in volume. The false increases occur if a sub-atmospheric pressure is used in the collecting system. There is therefore obviously good reason to spend some time on this subject.

Sources of error in measuring gas volume for the assessment of ventilation

Temperature and humidity

The volume of a gas increases if it is heated or its pressure reduced. The volume will be diminished if humidity, or water vapour pressure, is increased. The influence of temperature and humidity on gas volume is given in Table 13.1. To give an example, this means that room air at 20°C and a relative humidity of 50% (corresponding to P_{H_2O} of 1·2 kPa (9 mm Hg) at a barometric pressure of 760 mm Hg) expands when heated to body temperature (37°C) and slightly decreases in volume with a simultaneous increase in humidity which is 100% in the lung (P_{H_2O} of 6·25 kPa or 47 mm Hg). Overall, the volume increases. When expired, the volume is again reduced from what it was in the lung. To measure the volume or ventilation inside the lung, it is necessary either to maintain the

Table 13.1   Factors influencing gas volume measurement

Factor	Influence
Temperature	0·37%/°C
Humidity	0·07%/% relative humidity
Pressure	
Inspiration	0·1%/cm H_2O
Expiration	0.1%/unit compressible volume per cm H_2O

79

expired gas at body temperature and 100% water saturation until its volume has been measured, or to correct the volume that was measured at ambient temperature and humidity back to body temperature and saturated with water vapour. This is achieved by using the BTPS factor (**body** tem-perature, **p**ressure **s**aturated (with water vapour)) which is given in Table 13.2. Under the given conditions, the BTPS factor will be 1·09 which is used as a standard factor when converting gas volume from ambient to body temperature and saturated water vapour. For a patient with a fever of 40°C, the BTPS factor is higher—1·11. The difference is, however, just 2%, and a varied BTPS factor is seldom used in practice.

Pressure

If the ventilation is conducted by means of positive pressure, as with most ventilators, the inspired gas will be compressed. If measured during increased airway pressure, the volume will be smaller than if measured at atmospheric pressure. The decrease in volume can be deducted by Boyle's law if constant temperature is assumed, as given in Tables 13.1 and 13.2. To give an example, inserting 10 cm H_2O for the change in pressure (ΔP) and

Table 13.2   Conversion factors for gas volumes, from ATPS to BTPS

Derivation of conversion factor:

$$V_{BTPS} = V_{ATPS} \left(\frac{273+37}{273+t} \right) \left(\frac{P_B - P_{H_2O}}{P_B - 6\cdot3} \right) \tag{1}$$

Where P_B = barometric pressure; P_{H_2O} = water vapour pressure at ambient temperature; t = ambient temperature; $6\cdot3$ = water vapour pressure (in kPa; = 47 mm Hg) at standard body temperature (37°C).

Conversion (from ATPD to BTPS) factor at different ambient temperature

Ambient temperature (°C)	Conversion factor	Saturated water vapour pressure	
		(kPa)	(mm Hg)
15	1·129	1·71	12·8
16	1·124	1·81	13·6
17	1·119	1·93	14·5
18	1·113	2·07	15·5
19	1·108	2·20	16·5
20	1·103	2·33	17·5
21	1·097	2·48	18·6
22	1·092	2·64	19·8
23	1·086	2·80	21·0
24	1·081	2·99	22·4
25	1·075	3·16	23·7
26	1·069	3·66	25·2

assuming a barometric pressure of 1033 cm H_2O (760 mm Hg), the volume decrease is 0·97% or, rounded off, 1%. The influence is obviously small, but can account for a 3–4% underestimation of ventilation in conditions where mean inspiratory airway pressure is 30–40 cm H_2O, if ventilation is measured with a gas flowmeter inserted into the inspiratory tubing. There will, however, be no underestimation if ventilation is measured in the expiratory tubing, because flow or volume is measured after pressure release to atmospheric pressure. If a PEEP device has been applied after the flow/volume meter, it will cause an underestimation of expired ventilation in proportion to the PEEP (positive end expiratory pressure) level, mostly only 1% or less.

Another and often more important effect of an increase in airway pressure is the compression of gas that takes place in the ventilator, tubings, and any humidifier and CO_2 absorber that may be in the respiratory circuit. Using Boyle's law, it can be seen that, for each litre of gas within the ventilatory system, 1 ml of gas will be compressed per litre of gas in the system per centimetre H_2O pressure increase. The pressure that counts is the end inspiratory pressure, because it determines how much is compressed in the ventilatory system when expiration is to start. If the volume of the system is 2 litres (assuming that a CO_2 absorber or a humidifier is in the system) and end inspiratory pressure is 30 cm H_2O, then 60 ml of gas will be compressed in the ventilatory system per breath, and 1·2 l/min if respiratory frequency is 20/min. If ventilation is measured within the ventilator, then the volume that has been compressed in the ventilatory system will be included in the measured minute ventilation, even though it was never in the patient. Knowing the volume in which gas can be compressed, however, a correction can be made for the measured ventilation. This could easily be implemented in a modern ventilator already equipped with the software for other purposes. Another approach is to measure ventilation near the patient, for example, using a pneumotachograph at the tracheal tube; then this error ceases to exist.

Finally, if ventilation is measured by gas flowmeter, it must have been calibrated for specific gases, for example, air. It may then give erroneous values if the patient is ventilated with another gas or mixture of gases. This can be appreciated by looking at Poiseuille's law which can be applied to laminar gas flow:

$$P = \dot{V} \times (8 \times \eta \times l)/(\pi \times r^4)$$

where P = driving pressure for gas flow, $\dot{V}$ = gas flow, η = viscosity of gas, l = length of airway, r = airway radius.

It can be seen that airway radius is of utmost importance and the airway length has less influence on resistance. What is of importance here, however, is that viscosity has an effect on the pressure drop in the airway. The difference between gases is small but can cause errors of 3–4%. Also,

Table 13.3   Sources of error in the recording of volume and ventilation

Source of error	Consequences
Leak	Can cause underestimation (positive pressure ventilation)
	Can cause overestimation (ventilation with subatmospheric pressure in respiratory tubings)
Over-range—too high flow	Mostly overestimation
Under-range—below scale	Mostly underestimation
Asymmetry of flow device	Different values for inspiratory and expiratory flows and volumes
Zero drift/unstable integrator	Increasing or decreasing end expiratory/end inspiratory volume

the viscosity is temperature dependent, but the effect on flow and volume recording will again be small.

All in all, the errors described so far can add up to as much as 20% of the true value.

Equipment for the recording of ventilation

Even larger errors can be caused by faulty equipment, erroneous calibration, and inappropriate use (Table 13.3). There is some discussion here about choice of the right equipment and performing a reliable calibration.

The most foolproof technique for measuring ventilation, in the author's opinion, is still the collection of expired gas, breath by breath, in a large spirometer that may accommodate 100 litres or more (so called Tissot spirometer) or in a large, gas tight bag (for example, a rubber coated Douglas bag) which is emptied through a precision gasometer. If the temperature in the spirometer or bag and relative humidity are known, a BTPS correction can be made. Although it is difficult to see how the calibration of the spirometer would change, the gasometer may deteriorate over time and therefore requires intermittent calibration. The simplest and most accurate tool to use is a giant syringe of at least 3 litres. Although simple in appearance, it is quite expensive, but is well worth it.

Even emptying of a rubber or plastic bag can cause a problem. Although it may not matter much if the bag contained 100 litres, it can cause considerable error if the bag contains just 1 litre, for example, in recording the ventilation of a neonate. This is because suctioning gas out of the bag will cause a subatmospheric pressure in the tubings and valves that connect the bag to the pump. If the gasometer is between the bag and the pump, its gas will also be decompressed at the end of emptying. If the pump sucks down to a pressure of −20 cm H_2O and the total volume between bag and pump is 5 litres (a reasonable value) with the gasometer near the pump, 0·1 litre will be sucked out by rarefaction of the gas, causing a 10%

overestimate in the neonatal case. By terminating the emptying of the bag at a less "negative" pressure, connecting the bag and pump with a small volume tubing, and placing the gasometer after the pump, the error is minimised, as is the case if the bag is emptied manually by compressing it.

As a result of the advantages offered by a spirometer–gasometer system, that is, being insensitive to pressure (except for the note made above), and the viscosity and density of the gas being easy to calibrate, it should be considered in experiments where the airflow curve during respiration is not needed, or as an additional technique for volume recording over time.

More common today is the recording of ventilation by airflow measurement and integration of flow over time to yield volume. Although simple to use, and often offered as a self calibrated black box, some or all of the errors mentioned above apply. Thus, it is common to use a differential pressure technique with a flow resistance inserted in the respiratory tubing. The pressure drop over the resistance is measured, and through knowledge of the pressure–flow relationship the flow can be calculated. It is not necessary that the resistance obeys Poiseuille's law which would require a laminar flow. If flow becomes turbulent at some point, it can obviously be accounted for if the pressure–flow relationship has been defined. This relationship is, however, affected by the gas composition (density and viscosity) and, if humid air is cooled, it may cause condensation of water on the resistance, so that its pressure–flow relationship is altered. The first series can be accounted for if calibration is made with the same gas as used for the ventilation, and the second can be avoided if the resistance is heated. This is the case for the Fleisch flowmeters which are commercially available.

Other techniques of measuring flow are based on: (1) the creation of vortices by placing a rod in the gas stream, each vortex corresponding to a certain volume of gas that has passed the rod (vortex meters); (2) pushing a "flag" in the gas stream which will depend on the pressure exerted on the "flag", but that will essentially be independent of the gas composition; (3) cooling of a thermistor in the airway tubing which will depend not only on the amount of gas passing and cooling the thermistor, but also on the temperature of the gas and its heat conductivity (humidity); and (4) fluidistor principle (oscillation of airflow in a symmetrical, double channel flowmeter).[1] All flowmeters have a limited range where they can be used. When designed for a low flow, they will exert too much resistance at high flow and, when designed for high flow, they will be too insensitive at low flow.

If the flowmeter is used for unidirectional flow recording, the pneumatic design can be optimised, within the limits of the measuring principles. If the flowmeter is used for bidirectional flow measurement, for example, when connected to the mouthpiece, it is important to ensure similar flow–pressure characteristics in both directions, otherwise one may notice, erroneously, that inspired flow is larger than expired, or the opposite. This can be prevented by taking care in connecting the flowmeter to the mouthpiece, valves, and tubings so that symmetry is ensured, and by checking the result by calibration of flow in both directions.

Another difficulty with flow recording devices becomes evident when the flow is integrated over time to give volume. The integrating procedure is dependent on a reliable zero flow signal, because any departure from it will be included in the integration process and add to the calculated volume. In earlier analogue instruments, a zero drift was a more or less consistent problem, making integration over several breaths a nuisance. With digital techniques, zero drift is less prominent but still a problem to be aware of. It is almost common practice in commercial devices to zero the integrator after each breath to avoid a drifting baseline. It precludes, however, the use of the tool to follow changes in the expiratory level over time. If the breath by breath zeroing is offset, a drifting baseline must be carefully checked for.

Ventilation measured by body surface sensors

The respiratory movements by the chest and abdomen (the second reflecting the excursions of the diaphragm) can be measured and translated into volume displacement in and out of the lung. This approach offers the advantage of being completely non-invasive and does not require any mouthpiece or facemask. It can be valuable during long term recording of ventilation in an awake subject. Moreover, it enables the partitioning of ventilation into a rib cage and an abdomen component. For example, a failing diaphragm can be detected, as can a paradoxical movement of the chest wall. Thus, in respiratory fatigue, an inward movement of the abdomen may be seen simultaneously with an outward displacement of the rib cage.[2] Such asynchrony increases the burden on the respiratory muscles even more, because the ventilatory demand will be increased to compensate for the decrease in net ventilation. Shifts in the end expiratory position of the rib cage and the diaphragm (abdomen) can be followed, as well as their individual movements, during exercise, sleep, anaesthesia, after surgery, in neuromuscular disorders, and in any other condition that might be of interest.

The recording of one of the two levels, rib cage and abdomen, is not enough for a reasonably accurate volume measurement, because the contribution by the rib cage and the diaphragm may change after the calibration of the equipment, and calibration has to be done in each patient, as described below. A single level recording can of course be used if the purpose is just to follow the respiratory frequency and detect any apnoea.

There are basically three different methods available for assessing the thoracoabdominal excursions: (1) magnetometry, (2) strain gauge technique, and (3) respiratory inductive plethysmography. Magnetometry was introduced in 1972 by Konno and Mead[3] and uses two pairs of electrical coils. One pair is positioned anteriorly and posteriorly on the chest, at the mammillary level, the other pair on the front and back of the abdomen, at the umbilical level. An electric current passes through one coil in each pair, causing an electromagnetic field. The other coil in the pair is moving in that field and creates an electromotive force which can be detected as a weak current in that coil. The electromotor force varies by the square of the radial motion in the electromagnetic field. For practical purposes, the limited distance the coils will move in a sagittal plane can be approximated as linear to the electrical output. This method measures changes in the anterior–posterior, or sagittal, plane. As the transverse diameter does not change to any great extent during normal breathing, and the rib cage and the abdomen mostly behave as though they have only one degree of freedom, the variation in the sagittal diameter can be used for volume measurement. More sophisticated equipment with four pairs of coils has also been developed, to enable both sagittal and transverse measurements.

The strain gauge technique has frequently been used in the measurement of variations in leg and arm diameters for the estimation of regional blood flow, but can also be applied for breathing measurements.[4] Rubber bands filled with mercury are wrapped around the chest and abdomen at the same level as the magnetometers. With a suitable baseline tension of the rubber bands, an inspiratory movement can be detected by the increased resistance to an electric current caused by the narrowing and lengthening of the rubber band. By this means, changes in the circumference of the thorax and the abdomen are detected. Thus, a change in the transverse plane in any direction will affect the recording, contrary to what can be detected by the magnetometers. The strain gauges can, however, easily stick to the skin, or roll along the body, so that variations in the resistance of the strain gauge may not reflect the tidal excursions.

Finally, the most modern technique for assessing ventilation from body surface movement is inductive plethysmography. It is based on two zig-zag bands of electric wire that are applied around the chest and the abdomen, as for the other two techniques. When an electric current is applied to the wire, the wire acts as a coil and establishes an inductive force, the strength of which is related to the area inscribed by the zig-zag wire.[5] Accordingly, this technique measures the variations in area of the chest and the abdomen during breathing, at the applied levels. In theory, it should be the most accurate technique of those described, and today it is the only commercially available instrument for respiratory measurement.

The respiratory excursions must be translated into volume changes to enable the calculation of minute ventilation. The calibration principles are the same for all three techniques. Two will be mentioned here. One calibration is based on an "isovolume" manoeuvre, that is, the patient makes an expiratory effort with his diaphragm against a closed nose and mouth, and allows his rib cage to expand passively.[3] He then uses his expiratory muscles to compress his rib cage, while allowing the diaphragm to be pushed caudally. The effect will be that the "expiratory" movement of the abdomen and diaphragm will be equal in volume, but of opposite sign, to that of the "inspiratory" movement of the rib cage, and vice versa (Fig 13.1). The simultaneous recordings of tidal volume and of rib cage and abdomen excursions will then enable the calculation of the rib cage and diaphragm contributions to the breath. This is a relatively accurate calibration procedure, but can be demanding for an untrained subject or a sick patient.

The other calibration procedure is based on the normal difference in rib cage and abdomen contributions to breathing in the supine and erect positions. In the standing or sitting position, breathing is mainly by rib cage

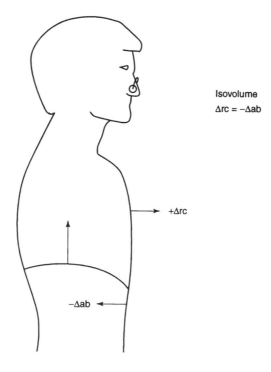

Isovolume
$\Delta rc = -\Delta ab$

$+\Delta rc$

$-\Delta ab$

Fig 13.1 The "isovolume" manoeuvre: calibration of sensors for detection of the rib cage and diaphragm movement and their contributions to breathing (for example, magnetometers, strain gauges, and respiratory inductive plethysmographs). Note that the subject is trying to inspire with his rib cage despite his mouth and nose being closed. This results in a cranial displacement of the diaphragm and an inward movement of the abdomen. The volume displacement of the abdomen and the diaphragm (Δab) are of the same size as that of the rib cage (Δrc) but with opposite signs.

movement. In the supine position, breathing is mainly by the diaphragm. If tidal volume (V_T) and rib cage (rc) and abdomen (ab) excursions are measured in both positions, two equations with two unknowns are obtained according to:

Supine:

$$V_{T_1} = (a \times rc_1) + (b \times ab_1).$$

Upright:

$$V_{T_2} = (a \times rc_2) + (b \times ab_2).$$

Assuming a linear relationship between V_T and rc and ab excursions, the equations can be combined and the constants quantified (Fig 13.2).[6] The advantage over the previous calibration technique is the absence of any complicated respiratory manoeuvre, which also makes the technique suitable in patients with severe respiratory disease, or in those who, for other reasons, are unable to perform according to instructions, for example, during anaesthesia.

A further simplification of the calibration technique is to record a large number of breaths in one and the same body position, because there is a specific normal variation in the relative contributions by the rib cage and

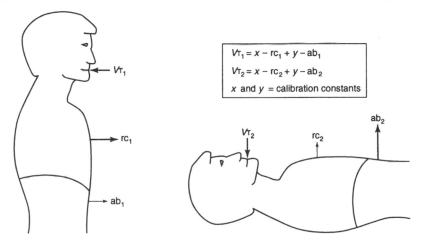

$$V_{T_1} = x - rc_1 + y - ab_1$$
$$V_{T_2} = x - rc_2 + y - ab_2$$
x and y = calibration constants

Fig 13.2 Calibration of equipment for the measurement of rib cage and diaphragm/abdomen contributions to respiration. Measurements are made at two different body positions. In the upright position the rib cage contribution to tidal breathing is larger than that of the diaphragm/abdomen. In the supine position, diaphragm/abdomen breathing contributes more to the tidal volume than the rib cage (in the normal case). If the tidal volume is measured, two second degree equations can be constructed with two unknowns. This allows calculation of the calibration constants for the rib cage and the abdomen contributions to the respiration.

87

the diaphragm/abdomen during "quiet" breathing.[7] With this procedure, the patient (or the volunteer) need not change position. This makes the technique applicable also in the intensive care setting (except when on controlled mechanical ventilation with no variation of the breaths).

Forced ventilation and flow–volume curve

The most common test of pulmonary function is the forced vital capacity (FVC) manoeuvre. After a maximum inspiration, the subject expires as fast and as completely as possible. The manoeuvre is a test of both available volume of gas and speed of expiration. It is therefore dependent on restrictive and obstructive disorders, the restrictive impairment reducing the FVC, and the obstructive impairment slowing down the expiration so that what comes out in a given time is less than normal. Common measures of expiratory flow are what is expired during the first second of the forced exhalation, the forced expired volume in 1 second (FEV_1) (frequently divided by FVC and multiplied by 100 to give FEV_1 as a percentage of FVC, that is, $FEV_\% = (FEV_1/FVC) \times 100$), and the maximum midexpiratory flow (MMF or MMEF), which is the midpart of the vital capacity, from 25% to 75% of FVC, divided by the time it takes to expire that volume (also called MEF_{25-75}).[8] Variables and symbols are explained in more detail in Table 13.4. These variables can be calculated on an ordinary recording of vital capacity against time, for example, on a Vitalograph. Modern spirometers are often flowmeters and present flows at given points of the expired vital capacity (VC) and present the recording as a flow–volume curve (or flow–volume "loop"), instead of a volume–time recording (Fig 13.3). There are theoretical advantages to doing this, because flow during the latter half of expiration can be reduced, compared with normal, before any other change in the spirogram can be seen (Fig 13.4). This is because the airways become narrower during expiration, and any obstruction will then become more evident than when the lungs are fully inflated and the airways maximally dilated. One can even say that the maximum inspiration is the most efficient way of concealing an airway obstruction, and that is the manoeuvre we use to detect it! The maximum expiratory flows at 50% and 25% of FVC are measured and called MEF_{50} and MEF_{25} (to make things more complicated, in American nomenclature these flows are called forced expiratory flow at 50% and 75% expired FVC, and abbreviated as FEF_{50} and FEF_{75}). The flow–volume recordings have poorer reproducibility, however, than the old FVC and FEV_1, offsetting some of the theoretical advantages of the flow–volume curve. Anyway, with the modern spirometer, you get them all—volumes and flows.

The performance of an FVC manoeuvre has been detailed in guidelines by the European Respiratory Society (ERS) as well as the American

Thoracic Society. The ERS guidelines are given in Table 13.5.

It was mentioned above that a restrictive disorder can be detected by a decrease in FVC. An airway obstruction may, however, also decrease FVC for two reasons: first, the forced manoeuvre will compress the airways as well as the alveoli. Gas can be trapped behind fully closed airways, and reduce FVC. With a slow "static" VC manoeuvre, the VC may be higher than the FVC because of less airway compression. Second, the chronic obstructions may close airways before a full normal expiration, even if it is conducted at low flow. The volume remaining in the lung, the residual volume (RV), is then increased at the expense of the VC. The reduced VC (or FVC) can thus be the result of either a restrictive or an obstructive disorder. The simultaneous recording of FEV_1 and flows will on the whole be a guide to distinguishing between these disorders.

Table 13.4 Symbols and variables of dynamic spirometry

Symbol	Variable	Comment
VC	Vital capacity	A maximum breath, from full inspiration to full expiration, or from end expiration to full inspiration
FVC	Forced vital capacity	A VC breathed in or out as fast as possible (can be smaller than VC in a patient with obstructive disease because of dynamic airway compression)
FEV_1	Forced expired volume in 1 second	The largest volume that can be expired in 1 s; will occur at the start of expiration, after maximum inspiration
$FEV_\%$	FEV_1/VC (or FVC, if VC has not been measured or is smaller)	Frequently used to assess airway obstruction. It can differentiate between restrictive and obstructive cause of reduced FEV_1
PEF (MEF)	Peak expiratory flow (maximum expiratory flow)	Must be preceded by a maximum inspiration because expiratory flow rate is lung volume dependent
MEF_{75-25}	Maximum midexpiratory flow	The volume expired during the midhalf of the FVC, divided by time
MEF_{50} (FEF_{50})	Maximum expiratory flow at 50% of the expired FVC	MEF_{50} is criticaly dependent on a full expiratory FVC manoeuvre
MEF_{25} (FEF_{75})	Maximum expiratory flow at 25% of remaining FVC	Note the American symbol FEF_{75} which describes how much of the FVC has been expired
FIVC	Forced inspired vital capacity	
FIV_1	Forced inspired volume in 1 second	Can be below normal in upper airway obstruction (for example, tracheal stenosis, paralysis of vocal fold, tumour)
$FIV_\%$	$FIV_1/FIVC$	Normally close to 100%, and thus higher than $FEV_\%$

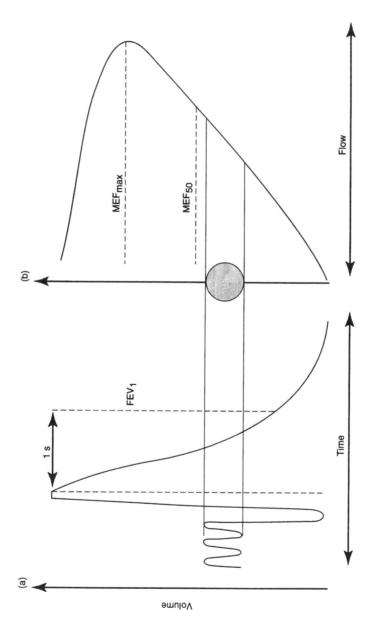

Fig 13.3   The forced expired vital capacity shown as (a) a conventional spirogram with volume against time and as (b) a flow–volume loop—recordings from a normal subject. Note the linear decrease in flow with decreasing lung volume despite the continuous full expiratory effort. This can be explained by dynamic compression of the airways (see Fig 5.4). Alveolar elastic recoil pressure will be the major pressure that causes expiratory flow and, as this pressure decreases with decreasing alveolar dimension, flow will decrease with diminishing lung volume. Note the early appearance of peak flow during expiration. This makes it mandatory that a patient makes a full inspiration before a peak flow measurement is made. Maximum expiratory flow at 50% of VC (MEF_{50}) is also shown.

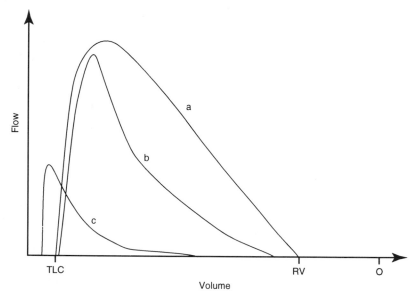

Fig 13.4 Flow–volume curves in health and obstructive lung disease: (a) normal loop; (b) moderate airway obstruction—note the almost maintained peak flow but faster decline in flow rate than in the normal subject; (c) severe airway obstruction—note the small peak flow and the very rapid decrease in flow so that, during most of the expiration, the flow rate is extremely low. This fits with severe dynamic airway compression and can be seen in emphysema. The increase in TLC and the very small VC are also findings that can be made in an emphysematous patient.

Table 13.5 Procedures for the recording of a forced vital capacity

---

1 If possible, a resting period of 15 min before the test
2 Upright posture, no tight clothing
3 A nose clip should preferably be used
4 A maximum inspiration with about a 2 second pause at TLC and then forced exhalation. The onset of expiration shall be as prompt as possible (the short end inspiratory pause allows stress relaxaton of viscous–elastic lung elements)
5 An acceptable manoeuvre should include maximum inspiration and expiration. The FVC manoeuvre should be performed without hesitation, resulting in smooth curves
6 At least three expired vital capacities with maximal effort. If eight forced manoeuvres have not led to satisfactory results the test has to be stopped
7 For the assessment of FEV_1 the starting point of the manoeuvres should be obtained by backward extrapolation to zero volume change of the steepest part of the volume–time curve. The extrapolated volume should not exceed 100 ml or 5% of the FVC. Alternatively, the starting point can be defined as that when flow exceeds 0·5 l/s. End of the expiration is defined as when volume change is less than 25 ml/0·5 s
8 The highest values shall be chosen even if it means that different values have to be taken from different recordings
9 If a measurement is to be repeated in the same patient at different days, the test should be done at the same time of the day in order to reduce the effect of diurnal variation

---

According to European Respiratory Society.[8]

91

A simple and frequently used method of measuring airway obstruction is the recording of peak expiratory flow (PEF—also called maximum expiratory flow, MEF). It is imperative that the patient makes a maximum inspiration before exhaling as fast as possible. The importance of this can be seen from the flow–volume curve. Flow reaches a maximum early on in expiration, and then falls continuously till the end. An incomplete inspiration will therefore inevitably result in a lower "peak" flow than after a full inspiration. This should be kept in mind when studying a patient who has difficulties cooperating, who is unable to inspire fully because of bandaging, who is in a body position that does not allow the diaphragm to be pulled down, who has pain when breathing, or who for any other reason cannot inspire fully.

The reason why flow decreases continuously during maximum expiration is that the driving force for flow is the alveolar pressure. The lung can be compared with a rubber balloon: the more it is inflated, the higher the pressure inside. This recoil pressure forces gas out of the balloon or the lung. What about the respiratory muscle effort? The expiratory muscles raise the pleural pressure which acts on the alveoli to push out gas. The pleural pressure adds to the elastic recoil pressure of the alveolar wall to yield the alveolar pressure which constitutes the driving force. If the muscle strength is maintained throughout the expiration, alveolar pressure will fall in parallel with the decrease in elastic recoil pressure, causing a decreasing flow. Moreover, the pleural pressure will act not only on the alveoli but also on the airways. At one point up the airways, as seen from the alveolus, the inside pressure has dropped corresponding to the elastic recoil pressure. At that point the pressures inside and outside the airway are equal and similar to pleural pressure. This point is called the "equal pressure point" and was discussed in chapter 5.[9] From that point and up towards the mouth, the airway is exposed to dynamic compression. This means that expiratory muscle effort will increase expiratory resistance and act as a brake during forced expiration! The net result is that most of the flow–volume curve is effort independent. A flow–volume curve looks much the same, at a given volume point, whether expiration is heavily or only moderately forced. It is only PEF that is clearly influenced by the muscle effort.

The relative independence of muscle effort makes the flow–volume curve interesting as a diagnostic and monitoring tool, even when the curve is obtained just over an ordinary tidal volume. It will give information about the behaviour of the airways, whether bronchospasm is developing, if oedema causes compression of airways, or if an increase in end expiratory lung volume by the application or augmentation of a PEEP prevents dynamic compression, to mention a few examples. To date, relatively little has been presented on tidal flow–volume curves in anaesthesia and intensive care.[10] It might be an interesting area for further exploration.

The inspiratory flow is less affected by chronic obstructive lung disease,

(a)

Subatmospheric pressure

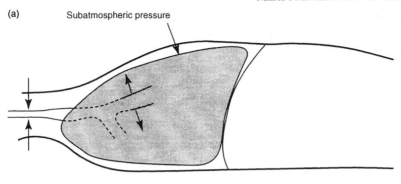

(b)

Positive pressure

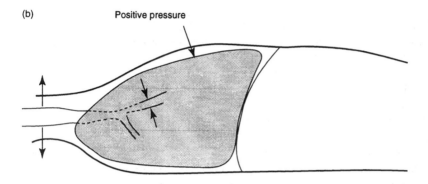

Fig 13.5   Dynamic airway compression of (a) upper extrathoracic airways during inspirations and (b) intrapulmonary smaller airways during expiration. Note that intraluminal upper airway pressure is subatmospheric in order to generate an inspiratory flow. This may cause intraction of the airway wall and the suctioning of soft tissue into the lumen. Intrathoracic airways, on the other hand, are expanding during inspiration because pleural and extraluminal pressures are lower than the intraluminal pressure. During expiration, intrathoracic airways may be subject to dynamic compression because extraluminal pressure exceeds that in the airway (see also Fig 5.4). Extrathoracic airways, on the other hand, have an intraluminal pressure that is higher than atmospheric and will be prevented from collapse.

because the airways are dilated by the lowered pleural pressure. Extra-thoracic airways may, however, collapse, or a loose part of the wall or a paretic or damaged vocal fold can be sucked into the lumen. This is because, during inspiration, intraluminal airway pressure is lower than atmospheric (this is what causes gas to flow towards the alveoli), so that the outside, atmospheric pressure acts to compress the upper airways. An inspiratory flow recording can sometimes reveal an extrathoracic airway obstruction by a lower than normal flow rate, whereas in the typical case the expiratory flow is maintained (Fig 13.5).[11] Obviously, this requires a spontaneous respiratory effort and can hardly be replaced by a mechanical inflation.

1 Hedenstierna G, Lundberg S, Rawlings D, Seeley H. Evaluation of a new spirometer based on a fluidstor technique. *Acta Anaesthiol Scand* 1976;**20**:7–19.
2 Sharp JT, Goldberg NB, Druz WS, Fishman HC, Danon J. Thoracoabdominal motion in chronic obstructive pulmonary disease. *Am Rev Respir Dis* 1977;**115**:47–56.
3 Konno K, Mead J. Measurement of the separate volume changes of rib cage and abdomen during breathing. *J Appl Physiol* 1967;**22**:407–22.
4 Hedenstierna G, Löfström B, Lundh R. Thoracic gas volume and chest–abdomen dimensions during anesthesia and muscle paralysis. *Anesthesiology* 1981;**55**:499–506.
5 Sackner MA. Monitoring of ventilation without a physical connection to the airway. In: Sackner MA, ed. *Diagnostic techniques in pulmonary disease.* New York: Dekker, 1980: 503–37.
6 Chadha TS, Watson H, Birch S, Jenouri GA, Schneider AW, Cohn MA, Sackner MA. Validation of respiratory inductive plethysmography using different calibration procedures. *Am Rev Respir Dis* 1982;**125**:644–9.
7 Sackner MA, Watson H, Belsito AS, Feinerman D, Suarez M, Gonzalez G, et al. Calibration of respiratory inductive plethysmograph during natural breathing. *J Appl Physiol* 1989;**66**:410–20.
8 Quanjer PH, Tammeling GJ, Cotes JE, Pedersen OF, Peslin R, Yernault JC. Lung volumes and forced ventilatory flows. Report of Working Party Standardization of Lung Function Tests, European Community for Steel and Coal. Official Statement of the European Respiratory Society. *Eur Respir J Suppl* 1993;**16**:5–40.
9 Mead J, Turner J, Macklem PT, Little JB. Significance of the relationship between lung recoil and maximum respiratory flow. *J Appl Physiol* 1967;**22**:95–108.
10 Brunner JX, Laubscher TP, Banner MJ, Iotti G, Braschi A. Simple method to measure total expiratory time constant based on the passive expiratory flow–volume curve. *Crit Care Med* 1995;**23**:1117–22.
11 Miller RD, Hyatt RE. Evaluation of obstructing lesions of the trachea and larynx by flow–volume loops. *Am Rev Respir Dis* 1973;**108**:475–81.

14:   Lung volume measurement

General observations

The measurement of lung volume makes up an important part of the functional evaluation of lung disease. Restrictive disorders have a reduced total lung capacity (TLC) with reduced vital capacity (VC) and often, but not always, reduced residual volume (RV).[1] A decrease in lung volume may not be the first sign of dysfunction but may reflect the progress of the disease, once lung volumes have become abnormal. Marked decreases in volumes can be seen in essentially all forms of acute respiratory failure[2] (Fig 14.1). Anaesthesia is accompanied by a decrease in functional residual capacity (FRC), so that it comes close to the awake RV.[3]

Obstructive disorders have initially normal lung volumes, but, as the disease progresses, FRC increases because of air trapping.[4] RV increases as an effect of premature closure of airways, and both FRC and RV may increase by an altered balance between lung recoil and chest wall tone; VC is reduced as a result of the inability to expire fully, compared with normal, and TLC may increase because of chronic air trapping and loss of elastic lung tissue (Fig 14.2). In the extreme case of emphysema, TLC may be markedly increased by several litres whereas VC is barely a litre. All the rest is an enormous RV that may be larger than the normal TLC. The lung volume measurement can thus enable a fuller picture of a lung dysfunction and, in the case of a combined restrictive and obstructive disorder, it may distinguish between them and give a quantitative measure of the severity of each. This may not be accomplished by forced spirometry and ventilation measurements; moreover, the recording of lung volumes allows for a more comprehensive analysis of respiratory mechanics which will be dealt with later.

Methods of lung volume measurement

There are a number of methods available for lung volume measurement. Three will be dealt with here: (1) gas dilution techniques, (2) body plethysmography, and (3) imaging techniques (*x* ray and isotope techniques) (Table 14.1).

Gas dilution techniques

By re-breathing a gas mixture that contains a poorly soluble tracer gas, the tracer will mix with the gas in the lung; its initial concentration will be lowered and eventually reach a new steady concentration. Knowing the initial and final concentrations and the volume of the re-breathing circuit, the volume of the lung can be estimated (see box). If the lung volume is the FRC, when re-breathing starts, it will also be the volume that the tracer gas is diluted in and that is being measured. If the subject is connected to the re-breathing circuit after an inspiration, then the volume will be larger and can be mistakenly interpreted as FRC. The re-breathing goes on until the tracer gas concentration has been the same for three minutes.[5] Termination that is too early will not allow poorly ventilated lung units to equilibrate with the gas in the re-breathing circuit, resulting in an underestimation of FRC.

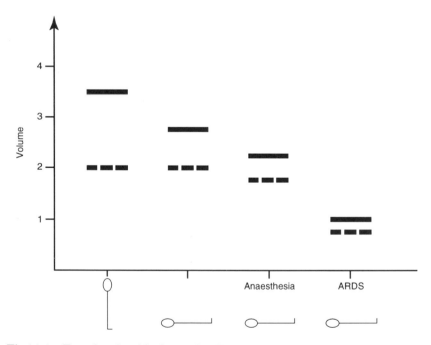

Fig 14.1   Functional residual capacity (FRC, —) and residual volume (RV, - - -) in an awake subject, upright and supine, as well as during anaesthesia and, finally, in a patient with acute severe lung injury (ARDS). Note the fall in FRC by 0·7–0·8 litre when lying supine compared with upright, and the further decrease in FRC during anaesthesia by another 0·4–0·5 litre. RV is unaffected by body position but possibly somewhat reduced during anaesthesia (however, as no spontaneous maximal expiration can be expected, the lung volume reduction has to be done by aspiration; the RV will thus depend on how forceful the aspiration is). Note also the dramatic decrease in FRC and RV in ARDS.

Although it may look simple, there are several details to deal with. Carbon dioxide is delivered to the circuit from the lungs and must be taken away by a CO_2 absorber. Oxygen is taken up by the lungs and has to be replaced by a continuous flow of O_2 into the system. The O_2 supply is adjusted to maintain a steady volume in the circuit, as assessed from the continuous recording of the level of a reservoir bag or a spirometer bell. There must be no leaks in the system. The temperature of the gas in the system must be read off at the start and end of the re-breathing, to enable correction for any gas expansion. The tracer gas used is often helium. Sulphur hexafluoride (SF_6) is another gas that has suitable characteristics. A schematic drawing of a re-breathing circuit is shown in Fig 14.3.

Another technique is nitrogen wash-out. It has been used relatively frequently in the intensive care setting.[6 7] As there is normally a steady concentration of N_2 in the lungs, it can be used as a tracer gas that is washed

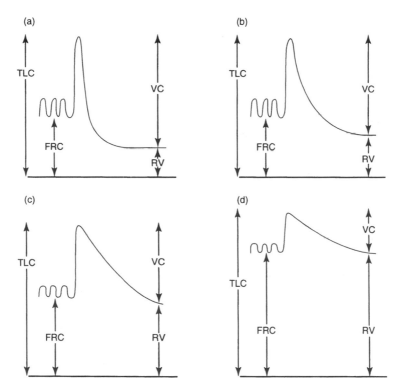

Fig 14.2 The evolution of forced expired vital capacity and lung volumes during the progress of obstructive lung disease. Note the slowing down of the forced expiration, the increase in residual volume (RV), and concomitant decrease in vital capacity (VC). Functional residual capacity is also slowly increasing as is the total lung capacity (TLC). (a) Normal; (b) mild chronic obstructive pulmonary disease (COPD); (c) moderate COPD; and (d) severe COPD.

Table 14.1 Methods of measuring lung volume (FRC)

Method	Principle	Comment
Multiple breath methods		
Helium re-breathing	Re-breathing of the poorly soluble helium until full mixing between lung volume and spirometer (steady helium concentration)	Requires CO_2 absorber in circuit and supplementation of O_2 to compensate for lung uptake (supplementation also necessary to keep gas volume of the spirometer–lung constant)
Multiple breath N_2 wash-out	Wash-out of N_2 in lung by O_2 breathing. Knowing the initial and final N_2 concentrations in lung gas and the expired amount of N_2, lung volume can be calculated	Less reliable if patient is ventilated with high fractions of O_2, because less N_2 can be washed out. Enables simultaneous analysis of gas distribution (see chapter 15). Some of expired N_2 comes from body stores and must be subtracted before the calculation of FRC
SF_6 wash-in/wash-out	Wash-in of a tracer gas that does not normally exist in the lung and then a wash-out similar to N_2 wash-out	Very low concentrations of tracer gas required (about 0·5%) which allows maintenance of the inspired oxygen fraction (of possible importance in the critically ill patient) may allow calculations during both wash-in and wash-out but can also be used for gas distribution analysis
Xenon wash-in/wash-out	Principle similar to that for SF_6 wash-in/wash-out	Xenon attenuates x rays which may enable regional volume radiographs (ventilation/distribution) measurements by repeated radiographs or CT scans; however, poor resolution. Xenon has anaesthetic properties
Single breath methods		
N_2 wash-out	An inspired VC of O_2, followed by slow expiration to RV during the recording of N_2	Easy and rapid to perform. Less accurate than multiple breath wash-out. Enables simultaneous calculation of airway closure and gas distribution
Helium wash-in/wash-out	As above but with 5–10% helium in the inspired gas	Part of the single breath CO transfer test. Less reliable than multiple breath techniques. Can be used with another tracer gas, for example, SF_6
Body plethysmography	Application of Boyle's law: subject in closed box, panting against an occluded shutter with the recording of airway and box pressures	Reference technique. Requires expensive equipment. Measures all gas in the lung, even behind occluded airways and gas in poorly ventilated regions (which may be difficult to detect with gas dilution techniques). Enables measurements in rapid sequence, contrary to gas dilution techniques which require new steady state concentration of gas before a new measurement
Imaging techniques		
Conventional chest radiography	Frontal and lateral views of the lungs	Gives qualitative information but does not allow any quantitative analysis
Computed tomography	Repeated transverse CT scans or spiral CT of the chest during breath-hold	Not a bedside technique. Enables regional volume calculations
Isotope techniques ^{133}X (or ^{127}X)	Similar to SF_6 wash-in/wash-out	Overall volume can be analysed by measuring inspired and expired gas concentrations, as for other dilution techniques. Regional lung volume can be calculated. Expensive equipment and radiation

out of the lungs by breathing O_2. The wash-out is terminated when the N_2 concentration has reached a low concentration—90% of the initial value or about 2%. The wash-out period and the final concentration will, however, be determined by the sensitivity and accuracy of the recording equipment and the homogeneity of gas distribution in the lung. Lung units with a slow wash-out require a long time to contribute to any substantial amount of the N_2. If the wash-out is terminated too early, these "slow" units may be missed in the calculation of the FRC, similar to the effect of a too early termination of the re-breathing procedure described above. During the wash-out, the expired N_2 can be continuously recorded. If multiplied by a simultaneous recording of expiratory flow, and integrated over time, the amount of N_2 washed out breath by breath can be calculated. Alternatively, the expired gas can be collected in a bag, or a large spirometer, and the

---

Equations for the assessment of FRC by multiple breath gas dilution techniques

Helium re-breathing

The spirometer and extra equipment, as shown in Fig 15.3, have a volume of gas (V_{spiro}) with a concentration of helium ($C_{initial}$). The subject under study is connected to the spirometer after an ordinary expiration to FRC. After some time, a few minutes in a healthy subject and 20 minutes or more in a patient with severe obstructive lung disease, the helium has equilibrated with the air in the lung so that a final, stable helium concentration (C_{final}) can be read off. Thus:

$$V_{spiro} \times C_{initial} = (V_{spiro} + FRC) \times C_{final}.$$

Solving for FRC:

$$FRC = (V_{spiro} \times C_{initial} / C_{final}) - V_{spiro}.$$

Nitrogen wash-out

The subject is breathing air or a gas mixture containing a known concentration of N_2 ($C_{N_2\ initial}$). After an ordinary expiration to FRC, he or she breathes O_2 with normal tidal breaths until expired N_2 has been lowered to about 2% ($C_{N_2\ end}$). During the O_2 breathing, expired gas is collected in a bag to enable the measurement of the expired amount of N_2 ($V_{N_2\ bag}$) which equals bag volume times the N_2 concentration in the bag. The expired N_2 comes mainly from the lung, but some gas has been dissolved from body stores ($V_{N_2\ body}$) and has to be subtracted in the calculation of FRC:

$$FRC = (V_{N_2\ bag} - V_{N_2\ body}) / (C_{N_2\ initial} - C_{N_2\ end}) \times 1 \cdot 09 - V_{app}.$$

The release of N_2 from body stores during O_2 breathing is time dependent, with more being released at the start of the wash-out than at the end. The following numbers can be used: 40, 35, and 28 ml for the first, second, and third minute of wash-out, respectively.[13]

volume and N_2 concentration are measured after complete mixing has been ensured (see box). Nitrogen may be poorly soluble in tissues, but there are substantial stores in the body, some of which will be washed out together with the N_2 in the alveoli. This has to be corrected for, as shown in the box.

If a tracer gas is used that is not in the lung from the start, it has first to be washed into a steady alveolar concentration. One example is SF_6. Despite needing a wash-in before it can be washed out, it has some advantages: the gas is practically insoluble in blood and tissues, so correction for body stores is not needed; smaller changes in gas composition are possible with SF_6 than with N_2, so that the inspiratory O_2 fraction can be maintained at an almost constant and high level, if necessary. The technique works with as little SF_6 as 0·5% in the inspired gas.[7] This makes the SF_6 wash-in/wash-out an ideal tool for FRC measurement in the intensive care setting because a high inspired O_2 fraction can be maintained. The technical set up is shown in Fig 14.4.

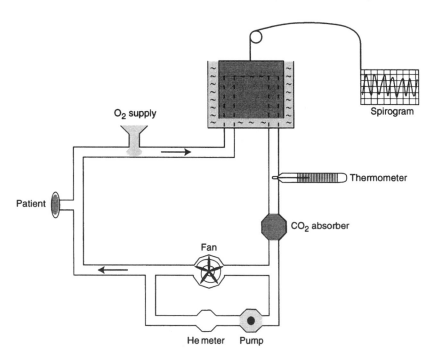

Fig 14.3   Schematic drawing of a helium re-breathing circuit. Note the continuous O_2 supply to maintain the volume of the spirometer system constant by compensating for the O_2 uptake of the patient. Note also the CO_2 absorber to scavenge expired CO_2 and the thermometer so that temperature related changes in spirometer volume can be compensated for. Finally, there is a fan to circulate the respiratory air.

The lung volume measurement can also be performed as a N_2 single breath wash-out. To ensure enough dilution of the N_2 in the lung, O_2 is inspired to vital capacity, after expiration to RV. This makes the test even faster, and allows other analyses of interest, which are discussed in chapter 15. The accuracy of the method is, however, inferior to the multiple breath test. The problem is that there is no single value for the alveolar N_2 concentration after the inspiration of O_2. The end expiratory N_2 concentration that is measured is weighted to the better ventilated units whereas the poorly ventilated ones contribute less. The mean alveolar concentration will thus be higher than the end expiratory N_2 level, but it is not possible to calculate accurately how much higher. It will cause an underestimation of the FRC.

Any of the techniques based on gas dilution requires a long equilibration or wash-out time to detect poorly ventilated lung units. If there are regions that are almost non-ventilated, as may be the case in severe asthma or

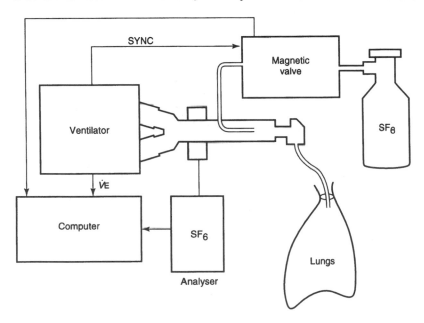

Fig 14.4 Set up for the online determination of SF_6 wash-in/wash-out for the assessment of FRC and gas distribution (according to Jonmarker[7]). As shown, the set up is used for mechanical ventilation, but in theory a similar set up can be made for spontaneously breathing subjects, provided that the dosing unit of SF_6 can be regulated by the inspiratory flow to keep inspiratory SF_6 concentrations stable. When expired SF_6 concentration is constant, the wash-out can begin. By online recording of SF_6 concentration and gas flow, the expired amount of SF_6 can be calculated and the accumulated volume during the wash-out can be used for lung volume determinations. The breath by breath change in gas concentration can also be used for calculating gas distribution indices (see chapter 15).

chronic bronchitis with emphysema, these regions will pass undetected, so that the measured FRC is an underestimation of the true value.

Body plethysmography

In body plethysmography, the patient sits in an airtight chamber or box—the plethysmograph.[8] He or she breathes through a mouthpiece with a shutter (Fig 14.5). The shutter is suddenly closed and the subject is instructed to breathe out against the occluded airway. By this means, the gas in the lungs is compressed which can be detected by a sensitive spirometer connected to the box, or by the pressure variation inside the box. At the same time the mouth pressure is measured and, as no gas is

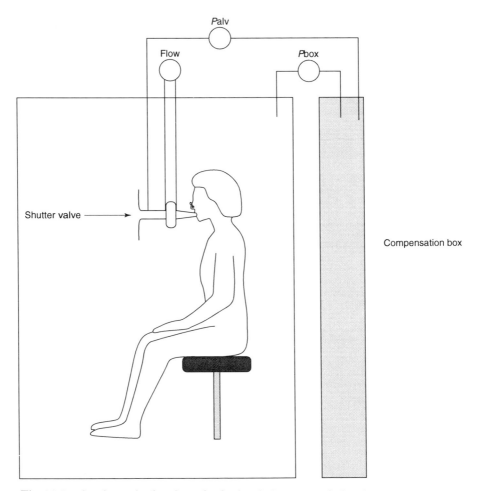

Fig 14.5   A schematic drawing of a body plethysmograph for the assessment of lung volume and airway resistance. Palv, alveolar pressure; Pbox, box pressure.

102

flowing out of the lung, the mouth pressure equals that in the alveoli. These variables can be used for determining lung volume by the application of Boyle's law (see box). Temperature is assumed to be constant. In practice, the subject is breathing in and out against the shutter, so that the lung gas is repeatedly compressed and decompressed. The variations in mouth (alveolar) pressure and in box volume or pressure are plotted against each other, resulting in a straight line with a certain slope. The slope depends on the calibration factors and the lung volume.

The recording of FRC takes only a few breaths, after adaptation to the plethysmograph, and can be repeated almost indefinitely with a few seconds between each measurement. This differs from the gas dilution measurements which cannot be repeated until equilibrium of gas concentration has been reached after a re-breathing or wash-out procedure; this can take from several minutes to up to an hour in patients with obstructive lung disease. Another advantage with the plethysmographic technique is that it detects all gas in the lung, whether or not behind a closed airway. This is because all gas is subject to the compression/decompression manoeuvre. The

---

Body plethysmography: application of Boyle's law

If a volume (V_1) is exposed to an increase (or decrease) in pressure, from P_1, to ($P_1 + \Delta P$), the volume will change by ΔV:

$$P_1 V_1 = (P_1 + \Delta P)(V_1 + \Delta V) \tag{1}$$

By rearranging:

$$P_1 \Delta V + \Delta P V_1 + \Delta V \Delta P = 0 \tag{2}$$

and

$$V_1 = -\frac{\Delta V}{\Delta P}(P_1 + \Delta P) \tag{3}$$

if ΔP is much smaller than P_1 then

$$V_1 = -P_1 \frac{\Delta V}{\Delta P} = \frac{-P_1}{(\Delta P / \Delta V)} \tag{4}$$

as V_1 = FRC, P_1 = alveolar pressure (= $P_B - P_{H_2O}$ at zero gas flow and open glottis). Then

$$FRC = \frac{P_B - P_{H_2O}}{(\Delta P / \Delta V)} \tag{5}$$

where ΔP = changes in mouth pressure during panting against the occluded airway shutter, ΔV = changes in lung volume (or plethysmograph volume) during panting.

disadvantage is that the equipment is expensive, requires careful maintenance, and is difficult or impossible to use in severely sick patients,
because some cooperation is needed. No commercial boxes are available for
measurements in the supine position. Finally, the technique may cause an
overestimation of lung volume because abdominal gas will also be included
in the measurement. This is of minor importance in most cases, because
abdominal gas is only some 50 ml in the normal case. In bowel disease, this
volume may be considerably higher—several hundred millilitres. The
volume of abdominal gas is, however, exposed to other pressure variations
than the lung, so the contribution to the measured gas volume is less.

Body plethysmography has been used in anaesthetised patients by means
of specially designed body boxes, allowing the patient to be in the supine
position.[9] The respiratory drive may thus be large enough to force the
patient to make a respiratory effort against the closed shutter. Things
become more complicated during muscle paralysis, when no spontaneous
breathing occurs at all. There is a study in which the lungs were inflated
with a known volume of gas with a syringe, and the net volume increase,
that is, after compression of the gas in the lungs, was measured in a
plethysmograph together with the increase in alveolar pressure. These
measurements enable the calculation of lung volume using Boyle's law. The
method is, however, extremely sensitive to temperature changes.[10]

Imaging techniques

Conventional chest radiographs may provide some information regarding
the aeration of the lung, but can hardly be used for any quantitative
analysis. The introduction of computed tomography has made such analysis
possible, although it is computer demanding and time consuming. A three
dimensional reconstruction of the lung can be made by repeated transverse
exposures through the chest, from the base to the apex of the lung, and then
to use an interpolation technique between lung cuts to fill in the gaps.[11] A
complete set of data, covering the whole lung, can be obtained with the
newly developed technique of spiral computed tomography. The patient
slowly moves through the gantry of the CT scanner during a continuous
exposure that may take about 20–30 seconds. This precludes the need for
interpolation techniques. With either method, a transverse exposure
through the lung is reconstructed in a matrix of picture elements (pixels),
usually 512×512. Each pixel contains information on the density of the
tissue in that pixel. The density is calculated from the attenuation of x rays
and uses a scale that is frequently expressed in hounsfield units (HU). The
scale starts at -1000 HU (air), with 0 HU for water and $+1000$ HU for
bone. The density of the lung in a particular pixel with an attenuation of
x HU is:

$$\text{Lung density} = (x\ \text{HU} + 1000)/1000.$$

Thus, if the attenuation is -800 HU in a pixel, a common value in well aerated lung regions, the density is $0\cdot2$. This value is the weighted mean of the lung tissue itself, blood, and the gas in the alveoli. The inverse of the lung density gives the "specific volume" of the lung (1/lung density). The density of the lung tissue is usually taken as $1\cdot065$, and its inverse is the "specific volume" of the lung tissue (1/lung tissue density).[10] Having these numbers, one can calculate the aeration of the lung in each pixel per unit tissue as:

Volume gas (ml)/Weight of tissue (g)

$=$ Specific lung volume $-$ Specific tissue volume.

In the example above with a pixel of -800 HU, the lung density is $0\cdot2$, and the specific lung density 5. Similarly, the specific lung tissue volume is $0\cdot939$. The pixel thus contains $4\cdot061$ ml gas/g lung tissue. If lung tissue density is approximated to 1, equal to water, the calculation can be simplified to a gas/tissue ratio:

Gas/Tissue $= x$ HU/ -1000

where x HU, again, is the attenuation value of the pixel. With an attenuation value of -800 HU, the ratio is $0\cdot8$, indicating that 80% of the pixel contains gas. Thus, four times more gas than tissue is found in the pixel, resulting in 4 ml gas/g tissue. The error of the simplified calculation is only $1\cdot5\%$ which might be acceptable in most situations. Knowing the pixel volume, the volume of gas in absolute units can be calculated. Finally, by summing all lung pixels, the overall gas volume, for example, FRC, can be estimated.

Isotope techniques can also be used for lung volume measurements. Obviously, this is not the primary goal when applying an isotope method in an experiment or in a clinical evaluation.

It can be obtained as a byproduct, however, together with regional distributions of ventilation and blood flow. The basic principle is to measure the total activity of a radioactive isotope in the lung by external detectors or a gamma camera, and to take a gas sample of known volume from the lung and measure its activity.[12] If the total activity is divided by the activity of the gas sample, the resulting number times gas sample volume gives lung volume. To allow re-breathing the half life of the gas must not be too short. Xenon-133 is the gas being used, although its gamma emitting energy is not ideal for the sodium iodide crystal in the gamma camera or scintillation detector head. The subject will not be dealt with in any more detail, because it is a demanding technique that is also regulated by law, and therefore not accessible to anyone with no special training and approval.

1 Schlueter DP, Inmekus J, Stead WW. Relationship between maximal inspiratory pressure

105

and total lung capacity (coefficient of retraction) in normal subjects and in patients with emphysema, asthma and diffuse pulmonary infiltration. *Am Rev Respir Dis* 1967;**96**:656–65.

2 Gattinoni L, Pesenti A, Avalli L, Rossi F, Bombino M. Pressure-volume curve of total respiratory system in acute respiratory failure. Computed tomographic scan study. *Am Rev Respir Dis* 1987;**136**:730–6.

3 Wahba RW. Perioperative functional residual capacity. *Can J Anaesth* 1991;**38**:384–400.

4 Pride NB, Macklem PT. Lung mechanics in disease. In: Fishman AP, Macklem PT, Mead J, Greiger SR, eds. *Handbook of physiology, the respiratory system*, vol. III. Bethesda, MD: American Physiological Society, 1986: 659–92.

5 Hewlett AM, Hulands GH, Nunn JF, Minty KB. Functional residual capacity during anaesthesia. I: Methodology. *Br J Anaesth* 1974;**46**:479–85.

6 Paloski WH, Newell JC, Gisser DG, Stratton HH, Annest SJ, Gottlieb MF, Shah DM. A system to measure functional residual capacity in critically ill patients. *Crit Care Med* 1981;**9**:342–6.

7 Jonmarker C, Jansson L, Jonson B, Larsson A, Werner O. Measurement of functional residual capacity by sulfur hexafluoride washout. *Anesthesiology* 1985;**63**:89–95.

8 DuBois AB, Botelho SY, Bedell GN, Marshall GN, Comroe JH. A rapid plethysmographic method for measuring thoracic gas volume: A comparison with a nitrogen washout method for measuring functional residual capacity in normal subjects. *J Clin Invest* 1956; **35**:322–6.

9 Westbrook PR, Stubbs SE, Sessler AD, Rehder K, Hyatt RE. Effects of anesthesia and muscle paralysis on respiratory mechanics in normal man. *J Appl Physiol* 1973;**34**:81–6.

10 Hedenstierna G, Järnberg PO, Gottlieb I. Thoracic gas volume measured by body plethysmography during anesthesia and muscle paralysis: Description and validation of a method. *Anesthesiology* 1981;**55**:439–43.

11 Rosenblum L, Mauceri R, Wellenstein D. Density pattern in normal lungs as determined by computed tomography. *Radiology* 1980;**137**:409–16.

12 Wagner HN Jr. The use of radioisotope techniques for the evaluation of patients with pulmonary disease. *Am Rev Respir Dis* 1976;**113**:203–18.

13 Lundin G. Nitrogen elimination during oxygen breathing. *Acta Physiol Scand* 1953; **130**(suppl 111):131–43.

15: Gas distribution

The distribution of inspired gas can be assessed by: (1) following the multiple breath wash-out; (2) studying single breath wash-out of a tracer gas; (3) measuring the ventilation of each lung or individual lobes by bronchospirometry; (4) studying the spatial distribution of radiolabelled gas or particles in the lung; or (5) measuring the variation of x ray attenuation over the lungfields during breathing. The principles of these techniques are discussed in this chapter, with emphasis on the non-radioactive methods.

Multiple breath wash-out

The resident gas nitrogen is most frequently used as the tracer gas in multiple breath wash-out investigations. Any gas that is non-toxic and poorly soluble in blood and lung tissue can, however, be used after a previous wash-in. The principles are the same for all gases. Here N_2 wash-out is described as an example of the procedure.

If a subject is switched from breathing air to O_2, the N_2 in the lungs will be washed out breath by breath. It is obvious that, if there are regions in the lung that are poorly ventilated, these regions will empty their N_2 more slowly than the well ventilated regions. Thus, the most simple measure of ventilation inhomogeneity is to measure the time needed to wash out the N_2 to a certain concentration, for example, 2%. The time required is, however, also dependent on the respiratory rate, tidal volume (V_T), lung volume, and dead space (V_D). The wash-out time is thus a measure that is influenced by factors other than gas distribution (Box A). To account for many of these interacting factors, the volume of ventilation needed to reduce N_2 in the expired gas to 2% can be measured and divided by lung volume (FRC). This is the "lung clearance index" (LCI)[1] (Box B). The size of the V_T and V_D still has an influence on the result, and this has stimulated further refinement of the analysis of the N_2 wash-out. One approach is to use a multiexponential analysis, described below.

If all alveoli are ventilated to the same extent, in proportion to their size, the wash-out follows a monoexponential decay. The monoexponential wash-out will result in a linear curve if the N_2 in expired gas is plotted breath by breath in a semi-logarithmic graph with time on a linear scale (usually the x axis) and N_2 concentration on a logarithmic scale (y axis) (Fig

---

Box A Factors influencing the efficiency of nitrogen wash-out by oxygen breathing

1 Functional residual capacity (the volume of gas from which N_2 is washed out)
2 Tidal volume (the volume used for repeated dilutions, after subtraction of dead space—see below).
3 Dead space (reduces the part of tidal volume that can be used for the wash-out)
4 Respiratory rate (if the efficiency index is time dependent)
5 Homogeneity of ventilation distribution relative to regional volume ($\dot{V}/V$) (what is aimed at by the measurement)

Box B Gas distribution indices

1 LCI = lung clearance index:

$$LCI = V_{E(2\%N_2)}/FRC$$

where $V_{E(2\%N_2)}$ = the volume of ventilation needed to reduce N_2 concentration in expired gas down to 2%; FRC = functional residual capacity.
2 Nitrogen wash-out delay (NWOD or pulmonary nitrogen clearance delay—PNCD). The index is based on the following relationship:

$$F_{An} = F_{A}init \times w^n$$

where F_{An} = the alveolar N_2 concentration after n breaths of O_2, $F_{A}init$ = the initial N_2 concentration (79·1% during air breathing), w = the dilution factor $((V_T - V_D)/V_A + (V_T - V_D))$. Here, $V_T - V_D$ is the tidal minus the dead space volume, and V_A is the alveolar volume.

In a lung with different compartments with individual dilution factors:

$$F_{An} = F_{A}init_1 \times w_1^n + F_{A}init_2 \times w_2^n + F_{A}init_3 \times w_3^n \ldots F_{A}init_n \times w_n^n.$$

The fraction of each compartment of total ventilated lung volume ($f_1, f_2, f_3 \ldots f_n$) and their dilution factors ($w_1, w_2, w_3 \ldots w_n$) will define the number of breaths that are required to wash out a hypothetical gas molecule from the lung (n_{act}):

$$n_{act} = f_1/(1 - w_1) + f_2/(1 - w_2) + f_3/(1 - w_3) + \cdots f_n/(1 - w_n).$$

The ideal number of breaths will be:

$$n_{id} = f_1/w_1 + f_2/w_2 + f_3/w_3 \ldots f_n/w_n.$$

The ventilation homogeneity, or efficiency, as defined by the NWOD index is calculated as:

$$NWOD = \frac{n_{act} - n_{id}}{n_{id}} \times 100 \ (\%).$$

15.1). If the alveoli do not wash out their N_2 at the same rate, then the wash-out is polyexponential with each compartment having its own specific exponential decay. The N_2 wash-out will be a curve in a semi-logarithmic plot, made up of the different exponential decays. When the faster compartments have eventually emptied their N_2, the last part of the wash-out curve is linear again in the semi-logarithmic plot, reflecting the wash-out of the slowest compartment (Fig 15.1). If this single exponential curve is subtracted from the major, composite curve, by an extrapolation technique, back to the onset of the wash-out, the new curve will comprise the remaining compartment(s). By repeating the subtraction procedure, all compartments can be identified. The resolution of the technique does not permit more than three compartments to be detected, and in healthy subjects only one or two compartments can be seen.

If there are two or more compartments, the wash-out is delayed. The amount of the delay depends on the differences in the size and dilution factor of the individual compartments. There are different ways of expressing this and one is the "nitrogen wash-out delay" (NWOD)[3] (Box B). The NWOD index is unaffected by the size of the tidal volume, but it must be kept constant throughout the wash-out. If the wash-out is monoexponential, the NWOD index is zero. In healthy subjects, the NWOD index may be up to 35% and higher values should be considered pathological.[3]

There are other indices based on the same principles as the NWOD index and they offer no advantage over that index. Another approach is based on calculating the moment ratios of the wash-out curve. It may be the most accurate method, but it is more complicated. The interested reader is referred to Saniie et al.[4]

Other tracer gases that should be mentioned specifically are sulphur hexafluoride (SF_6) which can be used in minute amounts (2% or less; see chapter 14) and can be detected by infrared spectroscopy[5] and non-radioactive xenon, which attenuates x rays and can therefore be detected on conventional chest radiographs or computed tomography (CT) scans.[6] Xenon wash-out is discussed later—"Chest radiography and computed tomography".

Single breath wash-out

The single breath wash-out can be analysed for many reasons. First, it can give a quantitative measure of the efficiency of ventilation, that is, the homogeneity of the ventilation/regional volume distribution. Second, it can give information about the phenomenon of airway closure through recording of closing volume and closing capacity. Third, it can be used to calculate the anatomical, or series, dead space. All three analyses can be made with a single breath N_2 wash-out, but other tracer gases can also be

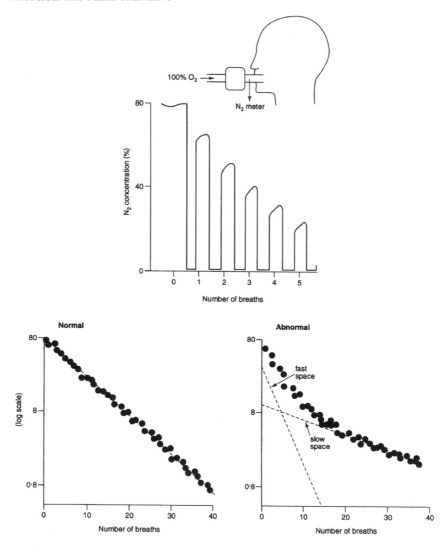

Fig 15.1   Multiple breath N_2 wash-out: (a) the technical set up. During expiration a three way valve at the mouthpiece is switched so that the subject is breathing O_2 while the wash-out of N_2 is followed. (b) In a normal subject a monoexponential wash-out is a common finding (note the logarithmic N_2 concentration scale (y axis) and the linear scale with breath numbers (x axis)). (c) A bi- or triexponential wash-out curve can be seen in a patient with obstructive lung disease. The wash-out curve can be partitioned into different components by a backward extrapolation technique. This means that a line is fitted to the latter part of the wash-out curve which comprises only one component because the faster one has already been washed out. By calculating the difference between the wash-out curve and the extrapolated straight line, the fast component can be obtained. (Reproduced from West[2] with permission from the author and the publisher.)

110

Table 15.1   Procedure for the recording of a single breath N$_2$ wash-out

Step	Comment
1 Maximum expiration to RV	Subject has been breathing air or gas containing N$_2$. No specific demand on flow rate during expiration
2 Maximum inspiration with oxygen to TLC	Steady rapid inspiration around 1 l/s or whatever is convenient
3 Immediate expiration (no breath-hold at end inspiration	An end inspiratory pause would enable mixing of gas of different N$_2$ concentrations and invalidate the measurement
4 Steady, slow expiration at a flow rate of 0·4–0·5 l/s	Too high flow will affect the emptying pattern between lung units and interfere with the expired concentration curve; too slow expiration will allow gas mixing between lung units and thus decrease concentration differences
5 Expiraton must be complete to RV	Incomplete expiration may make the calcualtion of the slope of the alveolar plateau less reliable, cause an erroneous, mostly underestimated, end tidal gas concentration, and cause an underestimation of CV

used, if they have been washed in until a steady state or equilibrium has been reached in the alveoli. In addition, airway closure can be measured by a slightly different technique, similar in performance to the nitrogen wash-out but conceptually different. These recordings are dealt with below. The procedures for a single breath N$_2$ wash-out are also given in Table 15.1.

Wash-out for the assessment of gas distribution

The distribution of inspired gas can be given a quantitative value by studying the change in expired concentration of N$_2$, or a tracer gas that has been inhaled to steady state concentrations. Again, the principles for a N$_2$ wash-out are described, but they apply to the tracer gases as well. Thus, if O$_2$ is inhaled, the N$_2$ in the alveoli is diluted. If distribution of the inspired gas is uneven in relation to the regional alveolar volume, then the N$_2$ concentration varies between lung regions. During the succeeding expiration, the "fast" or better ventilated lung units empty first and they contain more diluted gas with lower N$_2$ concentrations than the following "slower" lung units. This causes an increasing concentration of the N$_2$ during the expiration. The more uneven the distribution, the steeper the slope of the N$_2$ curve.[6] Thus, to create a sloping N$_2$ concentration curve, both uneven distribution and sequential emptying must occur. The sloping plateau can be seen during an ordinary expiration of the tidal volume. When gas distribution is measured, however, the recording is done during a vital capacity manoeuvre with inspiratory and expiratory flows at approximately 0·5 l/s. Flow must be kept constant at a predetermined rate, because it affects the slope. Also, no end inspiratory breath-hold is allowed, because it would enable diffusion of gas between lung units and reduce the concentration differences in the lung. The standard procedure is thus to

111

expire to residual volume, inspire to total lung capacity, and then immediately to expire back to residual volume. The expired N_2 concentration is recorded against expired volume, not against time.

Four different phases can be detected on the expired N_2 concentration versus time curve, as measured at the mouth (Fig 15.2). Phase I coincides with the expiration of dead space gas which contains no N_2, only O_2. Phase II shows a rapid increase in N_2 concentration and reflects the wash-out of dead space and gas from alveoli that empty early. The increasing alveolar contribution raises the N_2 concentration until it flattens off and increases more slowly. This flatter part of the curve is called phase III, or the "alveolar plateau". The N_2 concentration varies rhythmically as a result of differing contributions from upper and lower lung regions during the cardiac cycle ("cardiogenic oscillations"). Thus, the lower N_2 concentrations in the oscillating curve represent a larger contribution from lower, dependent regions, and are thought to be the effect of airway obstruction by the pulse wave when it is propagated through the major arteries in the hilar region. The slope of the curve is expressed as change in percentage N_2 per litre of expired gas. Normally, the slope does not exceed 2% N_2/l, but can increase tenfold in severe obstructive disease.

Wash-out for the assessment of airway closure

If the expiration continues, after a previous maximum inspiration of O_2, the N_2 concentration begins to rise faster again, and departs from the alveolar plateau, mostly causing a clear inflection point. This final part of the N_2 curve is called phase IV and is interpreted as closure of airways in dependent regions. The volume expired from onset of phase IV to the residual volume (RV) is called the closing volume (CV), and the sum of CV and RV is called the closing capacity (CC). The reason why the N_2 concentration rises when airways close in lower lung regions (basal regions in the upright position and dorsal regions when supine) is the fact that alveoli are smaller in dependent regions after a deep expiration (as well as at FRC). When all alveoli expand to TLC, they become equally large. Thus, the residual N_2 rich gas at end expiration will be more diluted in dependent than in non-dependent regions. When airways begin to close during expiration, the contribution of gas with lower N_2 concentrations ceases whereas the contribution of N_2 richer gas from upper lung units continues (Fig 15.3). This explains the sudden increase in expired N_2 concentration, as measured at the mouth.[8]

Another technique of measuring airway closure is based on the inspiration of a bolus of tracer gas, for example, helium, SF_6, or radioactive xenon. If the bolus is inspired from the RV, then it cannot reach the closed lung units, but is inhaled to the other, open units (Fig 15.3). When inspiration continues, the closed airways open up and air, which is now free from the bolus, enters the subtended alveoli. During the next expiration, air

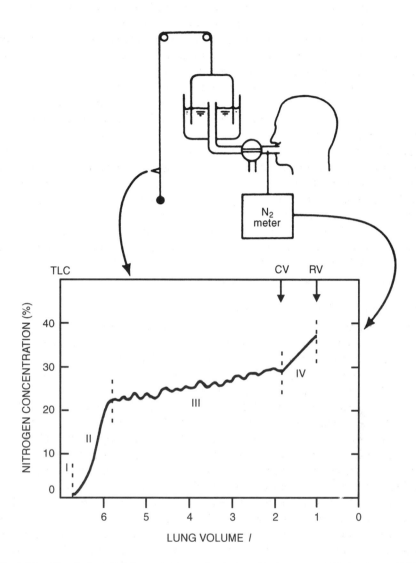

Fig 15.2 Single breath N_2 wash-out: after an expiration to residual volume (RV), the subject inspires O_2 to total lung capacity and exhales slowly again to RV. Note: the zero N_2 concentration at the start of expiration when dead space is washed out (phase I); the rapid increase of N_2 when the alveolar gas begins to appear in the mouth (phase II); the steady increase during the ongoing expiration and the oscillations caused by the beating heart (alveolar plateau or phase III); and the steeper rise in N_2 at the end of expiration, indicating onset of airway closure (phase IV). The volume expired during phase IV is called the closing volume (CV). (Redrawn from West[2] with permission from the author and the publisher.)

113

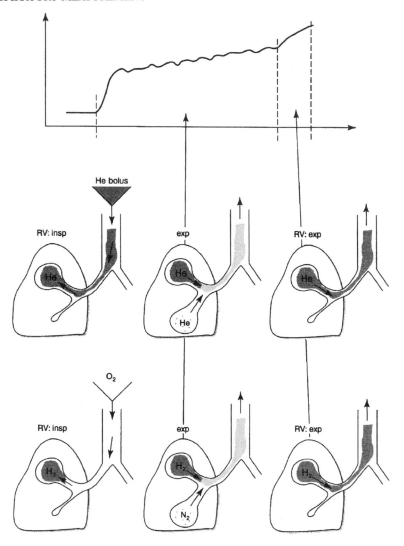

Fig 15.3   The principles of detecting airway closure by single breath bolus (upper panel) and O_2 techniques (lower panels). Bolus technique: after expiration to RV, the inspiration of a bolus of a tracer gas can only be distributed to lung regions with open airways. When, later during the inspiration, previously closed airways in dependent lung regions open up, the bolus has already been inhaled. During the succeeding expiration, gas from different lung regions is mixed in the upper airways, resulting in a certain bolus gas concentration at the mouth. When airway closure occurs, the contribution of bolus free gas ceases, causing a rise in the bolus gas concentration at the mouth. Oxygen technique: after expiration to RV, alveoli in dependent lung regions are much smaller than in upper lung units. An inspiration to TLC causes expansion of alveoli to the same dimensions all over the lung. Inspiration with oxygen therefore causes larger dilution of N_2 in dependent alveoli than in upper regions. During the succeeding expiration, the contribution of relatively N_2 free gas from dependent regions ceases when airways start to close, causing a rise in the N_2 concentration as measured at the mouth.

is emptied from all lung units, both with and without the tracer gas, and a plateau of tracer is established, similar to the N_2 plateau after an O_2 breath. At the end of expiration, the dependent airways start to close, and there ceases to be bolus free gas from these units. The other units with tracer gas continue to empty, so that the concentration of expired tracer gas increases at the mouth.[9]

Both methods give comparable results. The N_2 wash-out technique is, however, dependent on the VC manoeuvre to a greater extent than the bolus method. If inspiration is incomplete, the vertical N_2 gradient is affected and the inflection point, when airways start to close, occurs later during expiration, so that CV is underestimated compared with when a full VC is performed.[10] Also, if alveolar collapse is pending, a VC manoeuvre with O_2 may promote the collapse. The bolus technique is less dependent on the inspiratory manoeuvre and does not need extra O_2. On the other hand, the bolus technique gives information about gas distribution that is more difficult to interpret, because the expired tracer gas plateau is influenced by the inspired distribution of the bolus. Also, although the N_2 method enables a crude estimate of lung volume, the bolus technique does not (although in theory it should be possible, in practice the calculation of the end expiratory, mean alveolar concentration of tracer gas is too inaccurate). Thus, the choice of method depends on the situation for which it is being used. The N_2 wash-out may be the most versatile method for screening purposes, whereas the bolus technique may be the choice when CV is the only variable to study.

The CV is mostly expressed as a percentage of vital capacity ($CV_\%$), and is normally below 20%. There is, however, an influence of age with higher values in elderly people.[11]

Gas distribution (alveolar plateau) versus airway closure (closing volume)

It seems as if the CV may be more sensitive to airway obstruction in younger subjects, and in mild disease. When the disease has progressed further, the slope of the alveolar plateau increases and is more affected than the measured CV. This can result in part from the increasing difficulty in detecting the onset of phase IV, when the alveolar plateau becomes steeper. It is thus likely that CV is underestimated in more severe obstructive disease. The measurement of airway closure should therefore be considered a technique to detect early or mild airway obstruction, not for quantifying the severity in established or advanced disease.

It should also be mentioned that the expired concentrations of CO_2 and O_2, when recorded against time or expired volume, show a slope similar to that for N_2. The CO_2 curve has a more complicated origin, however, influenced as it is by both ventilation–volume and ventilation–perfusion ratios. It should therefore not be used as a substitute for the N_2 curve in the assessment of airway closure or the slope of the alveolar plateau.

Wash-out for the assessment of anatomical dead space

The single breath N_2 wash-out can finally be used for the determination of "anatomical" or series dead space. To this end a graphical analysis is performed in either of two ways.[12] One is to fit a line to the alveolar plateau and to extrapolate the line towards the onset of expiration, that is, to the left on the graph, as shown in Fig 15.4. Next, a vertical line is positioned so that it crosses phase II and creates equally large areas between the extrapolated alveolar plateau line and the vertical lines, and the N_2 concentration curve on one hand, and the horizontal zero line (0% N_2) and the vertical line and the N_2 concentration curve on the other. The volume expired up to the vertical line gives the anatomical dead space. This is the so called "equal area" or "Fowler's" method, after its inventor. The other approach is the "Langley" method, again named after the person who first presented the technique,[12] and is based on the extrapolation of a line fitted onto the accumulated amount of N_2 expired versus expired volume. Where the line intersects the volume axis, the dead space can be read off. It should be clear that the anatomical dead space that is measured by this approach differs from that calculated from expired and arterial CO_2 tensions, or from inert gas elimination, which will also include any alveolar, or parallel, dead space. This is dealt with later (see chapter 19).

Chest radiography and computed tomography

The variation in x ray attenuation during breathing can be used to assess the regional ventilation. The conventional chest radiograph allows only a semi-quantitative analysis and requires an experienced eye and is not dealt with further here. The CT technique enables a quantitative analysis. It can be used to follow, breath by breath, the wash-in and wash-out of xenon, according to the multiple breath principles described above. There are setbacks, however. Xenon has anaesthetic properties and causes anaesthesia at concentrations above 50% which limits its use in awake subjects.[6] The sensitivity for detecting xenon is also limited: 1% xenon causes an attenuation of 1 HU. Thus, a wash-in–wash-out of xenon cannot cause a larger attenuation change than 80 HU at most, which can be less than the variation of attenuation during normal breathing. During anaesthesia and controlled ventilation, however, the xenon technique can be an interesting research tool.[13]

A comparison can also be made of end inspiratory and end expiratory CT scans. The change in aeration can be used as a measure, and the formulae described for the calculation of lung volume in chapter 14 give the gas/tissue ratio.[14] The change in ratio thus gives the ventilation per unit lung

(a)

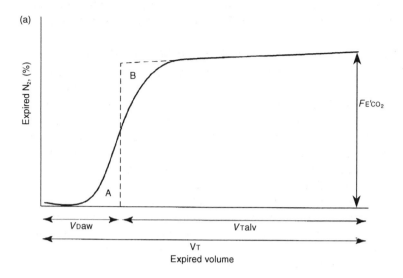

(b)

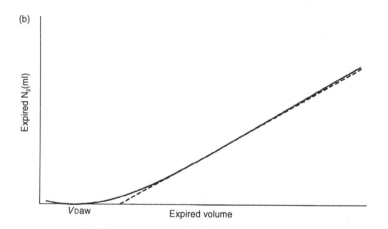

Fig 15.4 A graphical analysis of the anatomical, or series, dead space. (a) The "equal area" or Fowler's method; (b) the Langley technique. (a) Expired N_2, after previous inspiration of O_2, is plotted against expired volume. A straight line is fitted to the alveolar plateau and extrapolated towards the start of expiration. Another, vertical line is fitted on the phase II (steep rise of the curve) so that areas A and B in the figure are of equal size. The volume expired until the vertical line is considered to indicate dead space. (b) Accumulated expired N_2, after previous inspiration of O_2, is plotted against expired volume. A line is fitted to the N_2 curve and extrapolated backwards to the x axis. The volume expired until the intersection point is considered to indicate the anatomical dead space.

$V_D$aw = airway (or anatomical) dead space; $V_T$alv = alveolar part of V_T; V_T = tidal volume (sum of $V_D$aw and $V_T$alv).

117

tissue, or per alveolus. This is a standard way of presenting ventilation distribution and accounts for differences in alveolar size in upper and lower lung regions. This also means that, after correction for lung tissue, more of the ventilation seems to go to upper lung units than if no correction were made. This is an effect of the larger, but fewer, alveoli, and thus the smaller amount of tissue, in the upper regions. Thus, if the decision is made that ventilation should be presented as per alveolus, then the correction should be made. If the ventilation is just to be shown as it is distributed in the lung, and when relating it to structures or regional events in the lung, "uncorrected" values may be used.

Bronchospirometry

The ventilation distribution per lung or lobe was frequently assessed earlier before a lung or lobe resection. In those earlier days before isotope techniques took over, this was measured via a double lumen catheter, or a bronchial catheter, advanced down the trachea and into the main left or right bronchus. The ventilation of each lung, or an individual lobe, could then be measured. The resistance of the tube to airflow was considerable but rather equal between channels. The technique requires heavy sedation and analgesia of the airway and has become obsolete in clinical evaluations in patients who otherwise would have been awake and non-sedated. In anaesthetised patients, however, the double lumen catheter can still be used and offers the advantage of accurate recordings of individual lung ventilation.[15] This may not be sufficient reason to introduce the catheter, because its size may cause damage to the larynx and the airway wall, but it also enables the recording of the mechanics of each lung as well as individual lung blood flow by inert gas elimination technique, which is dealt with elsewhere.

Isotope techniques

The inhalation of a radioactive gas can be used as a tracer in a subsequent multiple breath wash-out, as outlined above. A suitable gas for that purpose is ^{133}Xe, or ^{127}Xe, which has a higher energy level and ensures better image quality. It is poorly soluble in blood and tissue as mentioned above, so that it stays in the gas phase when inspired. When the wash-in is discontinued and the wash-out starts, the gas and radioactivity obey the wash-out formulae described above. This enables calculation of the ventilation efficiency for the whole lung as well as for individual lungs, lobes, or smaller units.[16]

Another approach is to breathe in nebulised radioactive particles, for example, water droplets or carbon particles. The advantage of carbon particles is their minimal size, typically $0\cdot1-0\cdot2$ μm, which makes them behave almost as a gas (or a "pseudo-gas") with minimal sedimentation and impact on airway walls. Most of the particles will therefore reach and attach to the alveolar wall.[17] They are produced at the moment of investigation by burning a carbon rod, saturated with xenon dissolved in saline, in an electric high voltage circuit. The burnt particles are collected in a chamber and inspired. No wash-out procedure is needed or even possible, the particles being engulfed by macrophages and other cells belonging to the immunological defence system. The distribution of the radioactivity can then be measured by external detectors or a gamma camera, as for the radioactive xenon wash-out.

The ventilation distribution can also be studied during continuous breathing of krypton-81m (^{81m}Kr). This gas has a very short half life of 13 seconds which makes the gas fade on its way into the alveoli. The regional activity therefore reflects the ventilation distribution and not, or to a much less extent, the gas volume distribution.[18]

The radioactivity can be detected by a number of liquid scintillators (Geiger-Müller counters) or a gamma camera. The camera can rotate around the body and collect data in different angles which enables a three dimensional reconstruction of the distribution of the activity. The programme for these calculations is essentially the same as that used to reconstruct the CT scans. For further details on the isotope measurements, the reader is referred to more dedicated literature.

1 Bouhuys A, Lichtneckert S, Lundgren C, Lundin G. Voluntary changes in breathing pattern and N_2 clearance from lungs. *J Appl Physiol* 1961;**16**:1039–42.
2 West JB. Tests of pulmonary function. *Respiratory physiology—the essentials*, 4th edn. Baltimore, MA: Williams & Wilkins, 1990.
3 Fowler WS, Cornish Jr ER, Kety SS. Lung function studies. VIII. Analysis of alveolar ventilation by pulmonary N_2 clearance curves. *J Clin Invest* 1952;**31**:40–50.
4 Saniie J, Saidel GM, Chester EH. Real-time moment analysis of pulmonary nitrogen wash-out. *J Appl Physiol* 1979;**46**:1184–90.
5 Larsson A, Jonmarker C, Lindahl SG, Werner O. Lung function in the supine and lateral decubitus positions in anaesthetized infants and children. *Br J Anaesth* 1989;**62**:378–84.
6 Murphy DF, Nicewicz JT, Zabattino SM, Moore RA. Local pulmonary ventilation using nonradioactive xenon-enhanced ultrafast computed tomography. *Chest* 1989;**96**:799–804.
7 Buist AS, Ross BB. Quantitative analysis of the alveolar plateau in the diagnosis of early airway obstruction. *Am Rev Respir Dis* 1973;**108**:1078–87.
8 Anthonisen NR. *Report of informal session on "closing volume" determinations*. Bethesda, MD: National Heart and Lung Institute, 1972.
9 Milic-Emili J, Henderson JA, Dolovich MB, Trop D, Kaneko K. Regional distribution of inspired gas in the lung. *J Appl Physiol* 1966;**21**:749–59.
10 Holtz B, Bake B, Oxhoj H. Effect of inspired volume on closing volume. *J Appl Physiol* 1976;**41**:623–30.
11 Leblanc P, Ruff F, Milic-Emili J. Effects of age and body position on "airway closure' in man. *J Appl Physiol* 1970;**28**:448–51.
12 Fletcher R, Jonson B. Deadspace and the single breath test for carbon dioxide during anaesthesia and artificial ventilation. Effects of tidal volume and frequency of respiration. *Br J Anaesth* 1984;**56**:109–19.
13 Tomiyama N, Takeuchi N, Imanaka H, Matsuura N, Morimoto S, Ikezoe J, et al. Mechanism of gravity-dependent atelectasis. Analysis by nonradioactive xenon-enhanced

dynamic computed tomography. *Invest Radiol* 1993;**28**:633–8.

14 Pelosi P, D'Andrea L, Vitale G, Pesenti A, Gattinoni L. Vertical gradient of regional lung inflation in adult respiratory distress syndrome. *Am J Respir Crit Care Med* 1994; **149**:8–13.

15 Hambraeus-Jonzon K, Bindslev L, Jolin Mellgård Å, Hedenstierna G. Hypoxic pulmonary vasoconstriction in human lungs. *Anesthesiology* 1997;**86**:308–15.

16 Amis TC, Jones HA, Hughes JMB. Effect of posture on inter-regional distribution of pulmonary ventilation in man. *Respir Physiol* 1984;**56**:145–67.

17 Burch WM, Sullivan PJ, Lomas FE, Evans VA, McLaren CJ, Arnot-RN. Lung ventilation studies with technetium-99m Pseudogas. *J Nucl Med* 1986;**27**:842–6.

18 Fazio F, Lavender JP. [81m]Kr ventilation and ^{99m}Tc perfusion scanning for the differential diagnosis of pulmonary embolism. *Prog Respir Res* 1980;**13**:55–65.

16: Mechanics of the respiratory system: compliance

General

The two most commonly used variables for the evaluation of the respiratory mechanics are compliance and resistance. One and the same variable, however, reflects different parts of the respiratory system, depending on the way in which it is measured. It is therefore not sufficient just to talk about compliance and resistance, which occurs all too commonly, but also to indicate which part of the system is being studied. Measurements during spontaneous breathing and artificial ventilation are also different and, even though the same pressures and volumes or flows may be measured, they show the characteristics of different components of the respiratory system (Fig 16.1). This is detailed below.

There are other aspects to respiratory mechanics. The inertance, that is, the resistance to acceleration of gas and tissue, is mostly minor and can barely be detected in healthy lungs and during normal breathing; it can, however, grow and contribute substantially to the total respiratory work during rapid, shallow breathing. The total work spent on breathing is for overcoming the elastic forces of the chest wall and lung, the resistance to airflow, lung tissue and chest wall movement, and the minor component of inertance, or acceleration of gas and tissue. Finally, power is sometimes used to indicate the demand on respiratory muscles, or the motor in the ventilator, to generate pressure and flow. Thus, power expresses the instantaneous demand and work the accumulated demand on the muscles or ventilator.

Compliance of the lung

Recording of pressure

Lung compliance (Clung) is the difference in lung volume between two respiratory levels, divided by the pressure difference needed to keep the lung at these two levels:

$$C\text{lung} = \Delta V / \Delta P\text{tp}.$$

The pressure that keeps the lung expanded at a certain volume is the transpulmonary pressure (Ptp), which is pleural pressure minus alveolar pressure. With no flow and an unobstructed airway, the alveolar and mouth pressures are equal, so that the pressure measured at the airway opening can be used for measuring compliance. Pleural pressure can be measured using an indwelling catheter or a needle, but this is seldom done because it is risky. Moreover, recording of the pleural pressure is a difficult task. The pressure differs between the upper and lower regions of the pleural space, giving different results depending on the measurement technique used. The complexity of measuring pleural pressure can be hinted at through a short description of an accurate technique called the "rib cage capsule" technique; this requires drilling of a hole in a rib and exposure of the parietal pleura to the atmosphere.[1] The pleural surface bulges inwards because pleural pressure is usually lower than the atmospheric pressure.

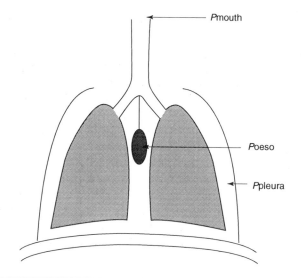

Component	Spontaneous breathing	Mechanical ventilation
Total respiratory system	–	Pmouth
Lung	Poeso	Pmouth – Poeso
Chest wall	–	Poeso

Fig 16.1   Pressure recordings in the respiratory system: recording site and part of the respiratory system that is being sensed.

Then a pressure is applied on the outside of the exposed pleura, so that the surface of the pleura regains its original position. The pressure on the outside is then equal to that on the inside. A translucent chamber is used to apply the pressure and to enable detection of the pleural surface. It is obviously not a technique to be used for clinical purposes!

The pleural pressure can be substituted by oesophageal pressure, which is measured via a catheter with a balloon threaded over its tip. The portion of the catheter inside the balloon should have several small holes, as well as an end hole, so that there is free communication between the lumen of the balloon and the catheter. The catheter size need be no larger than 1·5 mm internal diameter to ensure adequate frequency response, and the balloon should be 1 cm in diameter and 7–10 cm long. The catheter is on the whole swallowed easily via the nose, and is positioned in the lower third of the oesophagus.[2] The best way of doing this is to let the catheter be swallowed down to the stomach. On arrival at the stomach, it can be detected easily because the pressure swing is now positive during an inspiration. On withdrawal, the pressure becomes negative when the balloon has been pulled up as far as the oesophagus. The catheter is pulled out for another 5 cm, to ensure that it is positioned in the oesophagus. The balloon is emptied by asking the subject to cough and then reinflated with about 0·5–1·0 ml air. This volume should have been tested in advance to ensure that it does not cause any internal pressure in the balloon, and that the pressure remains zero (or atmospheric). Another test is to ask the patient to move his or her head in different directions.[3] Sometimes the recorded pressure increases with such movement, because the balloon is compressed. The catheter must then be swallowed a little more, and the test repeated.

The variation in oesophageal pressure during breathing seems to reflect the pleural pressure excursions when the subject is sitting or standing, but in the supine and lateral positions the mediastinal organs can exert a pressure on the oesophagus so that it no longer reflects the pleural pressure.[4] Thus, despite the many attempts to measure lung compliance in supine patients, these measurements are not as reliable as desired. The recording may therefore have to be limited to upright and semi-recumbent positions.

Procedure

Compliance is a static variable, that is, airflow should be zero at the two volume points, for example, end inspiration and end expiration. Measurements are, however, often made when there is no guarantee that flow is zero on measuring pressure and volume. To circumvent this problem, such compliance is called dynamic. Its value is limited, however, because it includes a pressure component to overcome resistive forces, and this component may vary from measurement to measurement. This pressure component can add to both the airway and oesophageal pressures.

Comparison of dynamic compliance values obtained at different moments may thus not inform on changes in compliance, but rather on variations in resistance. It could be claimed that, if pressure is measured at the moment when flow changes from inspiratory to expiratory, or vice versa, there must be a zero flow moment in between. This may not be true, because there may be a redistribution of gas within the lung (*pendel-luft*).[5] The breath should therefore be held for a few seconds to enable pressure equilibration between the alveoli and also between the alveoli and the mouth. In an anaesthetised and paralysed patient, it can be seen that the airway pressure drops rapidly during the first half second of a breath-hold, and then continues to fall slowly for another 2–4 seconds. This has been called "creeping" and may reflect reorganisation of muscle fibres and surfactant, rather than the elastic tissue of the lung.[6]

A suitable tool for ensuring a breath-hold is to close a shutter at the mouth. Another advantage is that it helps the patient not to close the glottis during the breath-hold which, if it occurs, would separate alveolar from mouth pressure. It does not matter if the patient is panting against the occluded shutter because the pressure will change to the same extent in both the mouth and the pleural space (or oesophagus).

Compliance is lung volume dependent. If lung volume changes between measurements, it can explain a possible change in compliance. It may be desirable, for example, in the fine-tuning of a positive end expiratory pressure (PEEP) to recruit collapsed lung tissue, but it can also cause erroneous interpretation of the progress of lung disease. In this second case, compliance should be measured at the same lung volume over time to enable comparisons, or compliance can be measured over seven to ten incremental or decremental volume steps, covering the whole vital capacity (VC). If the residual volume (RV) can be added, an absolute volume scale is provided so that compliance can be compared at similar lung volumes from time to time. Another way of taking lung volume into account is to divide compliance by the lung volume, to give the specific compliance. For example, if compliance has been measured over a tidal volume, it can be divided by the functional residual capacity (FRC) to yield specific compliance.[7] The compliance/volume relationship is not, however, linear (compare the pressure–volume curve of the lung), so a perfect compensation for a lung volume change may not be obtained.

To construct a pressure–volume curve in the anaesthetised and paralysed patient, an inflation–deflation procedure of the lung is needed. A suitable tool is a "super syringe" of bout 5 litres. In healthy lungs, inflation can be continued up to an airway pressure of 40 cm H_2O, and then deflated to a pressure of −20 cm H_2O in about ten steps with two second breath-holds in between. The procedure takes about 30–40 seconds. It is important to be aware that, as most patients have atelectasis during anaesthesia, a full inflation to total lung capacity (TLC) will re-open the collapsed tissue, at least if the breath is held at TLC for 15 seconds.[8] If the inspiratory manoeuvre is not to TLC, or the breath is not held for an adequate time, the atelectasis may remain. This should reasonably result in a lower compliance than if the whole lung had been opened up. The amount of atelectasis, and the expected effect on compliance, vary considerably between patients. No detailed analysis of the effect of atelectasis on the measured value of lung compliance has, however, been made as yet.

It can also be seen that the end expiratory level after an inspiratory–expiratory manoeuvre is greater than the end expiratory level before the manoeuvre. Thus, all the volume that was given to the lung cannot be recovered.[9] This may, at least partly, be explained by an ongoing O_2 uptake during the manoeuvre whereas CO_2 release is smaller with a difference of about 30–50 ml during the time it takes to do the lung inflation–deflation. The difference may be larger in a patient with increased metabolism, as it is in many intensive care patients. In these cases, vital capacity (VC) may not be larger than a litre, and the difference in inspiratory and expiratory volumes may be 10% or more of the maximum breath. Although a modest problem, it has promoted a lot of studies on how to do the pressure–volume recording in the intensive care setting and to establish a standard procedure. Heating and compression of the inspired gas may also influence the volume recording, depending on the technical set up. Finally, the time required to do the manoeuvre may be too long in a severe case of respiratory failure. A procedure that eliminates the effect of oxygen uptake and apnoeas is to increase lung volume by adding a PEEP of increasing magnitude every minute or so. At the highest level of PEEP, the tidal volume may be increased to make a maximum inflation of the lung.[10]

The recording of the pressure–volume curve of the lung (or the respiratory system—see below) may guide in adjusting the PEEP level so that the lung is moved up from a lower, flatter part to the steepest part of the curve (Fig 16.2). This should correspond to when the lung is fully, or almost fully, recruited. If the tidal volume is of such a dimension that an inflation is kept within the steep part of the pressure–volume curve, it is reasonable to assume that this is optimal in terms of avoiding baro-/volotrauma.[11]

Compliance of the chest

The recording of chest wall compliance is difficult in the awake, non-paralysed patient. The procedure requires a relaxation manoeuvre that only trained volunteers may be able to do.[12] Little is therefore known about chest wall compliance in spontaneously breathing patients with lung or chest wall diseases. In the anaesthetised, paralysed, or sedated patients, chest wall compliance can be measured together with the recording of lung compliance. The pressure that expands the chest wall (rib cage and diaphragm) is oesophageal pressure minus the pressure that surrounds the body (normally atmospheric, and set equal to zero in the calculations of compliance). Relatively little has been published on chest wall compliance, but it seems to be reduced in acute respiratory distress syndrome (ARDS), presumably as a result of general oedema.[13] It may add to the increased demand on inspiratory pressure in the ventilation of an ARDS patient. Similarly, the reduced chest wall compliance in a patient with severe obesity

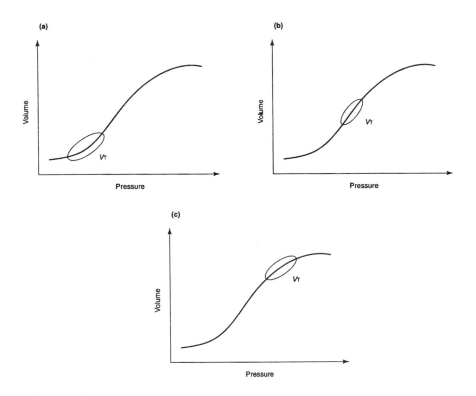

Fig 16.2   Location of the tidal volume on the respiratory pressure–volume curve at different levels of positive end expiratory pressure (PEEP). (a) Absence of PEEP causes tidal volume (V_T) to be located around the lower inflection point of the pressure–volume curve. This causes the opening and closure of airways and alveoli during each breath (increased shear stress). (b) A proper positioning of the tidal volume on the pressure–volume curve by suitable amount of PEEP. (c) Too high a PEEP causing over-inflation of lung regions.

may also increase the ventilation pressures, which may not, thus, reflect lung disease.

Compliance of the total respiratory system

Although it is not possible to measure total compliance in the awake patient, except for trained volunteers, it is the simplest procedure of all compliance measurements in the relaxed and anaesthetised patient (Fig 16.3). Total compliance (Ctot) is calculated as a change in volume (ΔV) divided by change in airway pressure (ΔP), under the assumption of zero airflow:

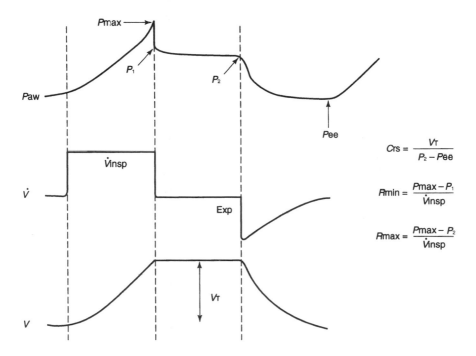

$$Crs = \frac{Vt}{P_2 - Pee}$$

$$Rmin = \frac{Pmax - P_1}{\dot{V}insp}$$

$$Rmax = \frac{Pmax - P_2}{\dot{V}insp}$$

Fig 16.3   The rapid airway occlusion technique during constant inspiratory flow. Note the rapid fall from maximum airway pressure (Pmax) to P_1 and the further slow decrease in airway pressure to an end inspiratory plateau (P_2). By dividing pressure with flow ($\dot{V}$insp) a minimum respiratory resistance (Rmin) is obtained, corresponding to the resistance in the airways, and possible rapid resistive components in the lung and chest wall. The division of Pmax minus P_2 with flow results in the total respiratory resistance which includes both fast and slow resistive components in the lung and chest wall, as well as any redistribution of gas in the lung (*pendel-luft*). A static compliance of the total respiratory system (Crs) can also be calculated by dividing P_2 minus end expiratory pressure (Pee) by tidal volume (VT): [VT/($P_2 - P$ee)].

127

$$Ctot = (\Delta V/\Delta P)$$

The zero flow must again be emphasised. Various commercial devices can be connected to the ventilator and, when fed with the airway pressure and airflow signals, they calculate compliance and resistance of the respiratory system. It is, however, more common to have a particular end inspiratory or end expiratory flow than in mechanical ventilation. This flow requires pressure to overcome resistive forces, but is erroneously included in the pressure required to keep the respiratory system inflated at a certain lung volume. The error thus causes an underestimation of compliance (and an underestimation of the resistance). This may in fact be why measurements of the respiratory mechanics are only of limited interest in the intensive care setting. It is not therefore too surprising if patients with emphysema (who have high compliance and resistance) cannot be distinguished from patients with fibrosis (who have low compliance and more normal resistance) when measuring respiratory mechanics.

There is a relationship between total compliance (Ctot) and its two components, according to:

$$1/Ctot = [1/Clung] + [1/Ccw]$$

where Clung is lung compliance and Ccw is chest wall compliance.

Intrinsic PEEP

In conjunction with the calculation of compliance, it might be wise to mention that any persisting end expiratory flow, just before the start of the next inspiration, signals a higher alveolar pressure than upper airway pressure—otherwise there would be no expiratory flow. This increased alveolar pressure is called "intrinsic" or "auto" PEEP.[14] It can be measured by occluding the airway tube for a second or so to allow pressure equilibration between the alveoli and the airway tube. Pressure must then be measured in the tube. Thus, an expiratory hold, which is a feature in some ventilators, can be used for the assessment of intrinsic PEEP (Fig 16.4). An alternative approach, which does not require any interruption of ventilation, is to measure the pressure in the upper airway at the moment an inspiratory gas flow is started.[9] If there is an intrinsic PEEP, no inspiratory flow will start until inspiratory pressure exceeds the pressure in the alveoli. Thus, by measuring the pressure difference in the upper airway between end expiration and the onset of an inspiratory airflow, intrinsic PEEP can be quantified. However, the technique requires carefully calibrated equipment.

Finally, the airway resistance can be calculated during inspiration (see below), and used to calculate the alveolar pressure needed to create the flow that is measured at end expiration. Again, there are limitations to the technique, mainly because inspiratory and expiratory resistances are not the same, and because resistance increases with decreasing lung volume. It is thus higher at the end of expiration than at any other point during the breath. Despite these limitations, it seems to be most important to measure intrinsic PEEP, which can climb to over 10 cm H_2O in obstructive patients. Intrinsic PEEP can also be seen in ARDS patients.[15] Uncontrolled, the intrinsic PEEP may be an unexpected cause of baro-/volotrauma.

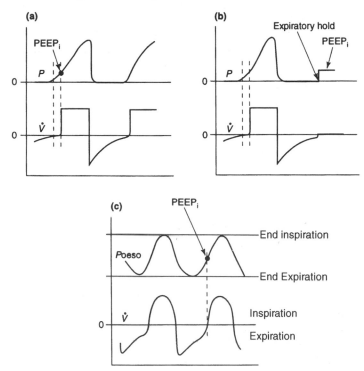

Fig 16.4 Assessment of the intrinsic PEEP (auto PEEP or $PEEP_i$) during mechanical ventilation (a, b) and spontaneous breathing (c). (a) Note that there is an end expiratory flow and that airway pressure has to increase to a certain level before inspiratory flow starts. This is because of an intrinsic $PEEP_i$ which must be exceeded by airway pressure before a flow can be created. (b) If expiratory flow is halted by occluding the expiratory outlet on the ventilator, airway pressure will increase as a result of the transmission of the alveolar pressure to the upper airways and ventilator tubings, corresponding to the intrinsic PEEP. It should be noted that, in the presence of a range of intrinsic PEEP levels (as can be expected in obstructive lung disease), the measured intrinsic PEEP will be a weighted mean of all values. (c) The detection of an intrinsic PEEP during spontaneous breathing requires the recording of oesophageal pressure ($Poeso$). Note that the inspiratory flow (Vinsp) has not started until a certain decrease in $Poeso$, corresponding to the intrinsic PEEP.

129

Compliance and atelectasis

Lung compliance depends not only on the elastic properties of the lung tissue, but also on the size of the lung. Thus, if part of the lung is inaccessible for inspired gas, whether through continuous closure of airways or collapse of lung tissue, then the measured compliance is reduced. In volunteers breathing oxygen at low lung volumes, shunt and a decrease in compliance were seen. These findings were interpreted as reflecting atelectasis formation.[16] In a recent study on the recruitment of collapsed lung tissue by a vital capacity manoeuvre, respiratory compliance increased after the recruitment manoeuvre.[17] Respiratory compliance, however, fell successively after the manoeuvre both in patients who did not develop atelectasis as seen on computed tomography scans (ventilation with 40% O_2 in N_2) and in those who did (ventilation with 100% O_2). The reason is not clear but the findings show that a change in compliance may be caused by many factors.

1 Olson LE, Lai-Fook SJ. Pleural liquid pressure measured with rib capsules in anesthetized ponies. *J Appl Physiol* 1988;**64**:102–7.
2 Milic-Emili J, Mead J, Turner JM, Glauser EM. Improved technique for estimating pleural pressure from esophageal balloons. *J Appl Physiol* 1964;**19**: 207–11.
3 Baydur A, Behrakis PK, Zin WA, Jaeger M, Milic-Emili J. A simple method for assessing the validity of the esophageal balloon technique. *Am Rev Respir Dis* 1982;**126**:788–91.
4 Van de Woestijne KP, Trop D, Clement J. Influence of the mediastinum on the measurement of esophageal pressure and lung compliance in man. *Pflügers Arch* 1971;**323**:323–41.
5 Hedenstierna G, Bindslev L, Santesson J. Pressure-volume and airway closure relationships in each lung in anaesthetized man. *Clin Physiol* 1981;**1**:479–93.
6 Van de Woestijne KP. Influence of forced inflations on the creep of lungs and thorax in the dog. *Respir Physiol* 1967;**3**:78–89.
7 Suter PM, Fairley HB, Isenberg MD. Effect of tidal volume and positive end-expiratory pressure on compliance during mechanical ventilation. *Chest* 1978;**73**:158–62.
8 Rothen HU, Sporre B, Engberg G, Wegenius G, Hedenstierna G. Reexpansion of atelectasis during general anaesthesia: A computed tomography study. *Br J Anaesth* 1993;**71**:788–95.
9 Rossi A, Gottfried SB, Zocchi L, Higgs BD, Lennox S, Calverley PM, et al. Measurement of static compliance of the total respiratory system in patients with acute respiratory failure during mechanical ventilation. The effect of intrinsic positive end-expiratory pressure. *Am Rev Respir Dis* 1985;**131**:672–7.
10 Putensen C, Baum M, Koller W, Putz G. PEEP-Welle: Ein autmatisiertes Verfahren zur bettseitigen Bestimmung der Volumen/Druck-Beziehung der Lunge beatmeten Patienten. *Der Anaesthesist* 1989;**38**:214–19.
11 Lachmann B. Open up the lung and keep the lung open. *Intensive Care Med* 1992;**18**:319–21.
12 Van Lith P, Johnson FN, Sharp JT. Respiratory elastances in relaxed and paralyzed states in normal and abnormal men. *J Appl Physiol* 1967;**23**:475–86.
13 Katz JA, Zinn SE, Ozanne GM, Fairley HB. Pulmonary, chest wall, and lung-thorax elastances in acute respiratory failure. *Chest* 1981;**80**:304–11.
14 Rossi A, Polese G, Brandi G, Conti G. Intrinsic positive end-expiratory pressure (PEEPi). *Intensive Care Med* 1995;**21**:522–36.
15 Tuxen DV, Lane S. The effects of ventilatory pattern on hyperinflation, airway pressures, and circulation in mechanical ventilation of patients with severe air-flow obstruction. *Am Rev Respir Dis* 1987;**136**:872–9.

16 Burger EJ Jr, Macklem P. Airway closure: demonstration by breathing 100 percent O_2 at low lung volumes and by N_2 washout. *J Appl Physiol* 1968;**25**:139–48.

17 Rothen HU, Sporre B, Engberg G, Wegenius G, Hogman M, Hedenstierna G. Influence of gas composition on recurrence of atelectasis after a reexpansion maneuver during general anesthesia. *Anesthesiology* 1995;**82**:832–42.

17: Mechanics of the respiratory system: resistance, inertia, power, work

General

Resistance is defined as pressure divided by flow $(P/\dot{V})$. The resistance to breathing is often divided into three components: (1) airway resistance, (2) lung tissue resistance, and (3) chest wall resistance. The airway resistance can also be partitioned into that of the upper and lower airways. In addition, a considerable resistance to airflow is often exerted by the artificial airway, such as the endotracheal tube and valves in the respiratory circuit. The recording of these resistances is discussed in this chapter.

Airway resistance

Pressure is required to force air through the airways. The driving pressure is mouth pressure minus alveolar pressure. Although mouth (or airway opening) pressure is easy to measure, alveolar pressure is not, at least not during breathing. There are two methods of measuring the alveolar pressure: the "shutter method" and body plethysmography.

Shutter method

One way of obtaining alveolar pressure is to halt the flow briefly and to measure the change in mouth pressure during this halt.[1] The pressure in the mouth will then equilibrate with that in the alveoli during the no flow period. If it is assumed that the equilibrated pressure is similar to that in the alveoli the moment before the occlusion, airway resistance can be calculated (Fig 17.1). The halt should be no longer than a few tenths of a second in order to avoid a deviating mouth pressure caused by the ongoing inspiratory or expiratory effort. Although this may give reasonable results in the absence of airways disease, the "shutter method" mostly underestimates airway resistance in patients with obstructive lung disease. This is because

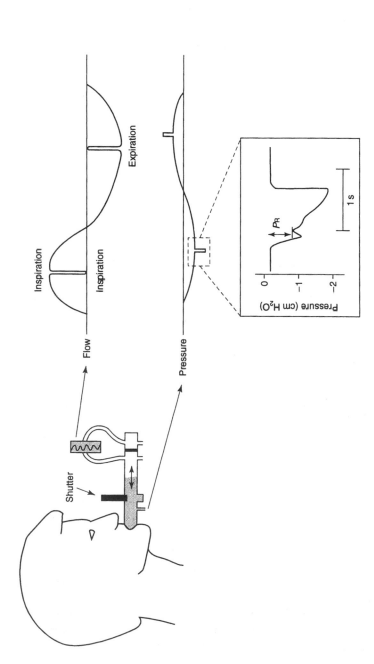

Fig 17.1 The shutter technique for the assessment of airway resistance (*Raw*). When airflow is briefly halted by a shutter at the mouth, mouth pressure increases during an expiratory manoeuvre and decreases during an inspiratory manoeuvre. This is because, during the no flow period, the alveolar pressure will be transmitted to the mouth. The mouth pressure will, however, also be affected by the ongoing movement of the chest, so that a biphasic pressure change can be seen, as shown in the insert. The rapid pressure change is assumed to reflect alveolar pressure, whereas the slower change is caused by chest movement.

there is no complete pressure equilibration between mouth and alveoli in the presence of airway narrowing during the short flow interruption. Moreover, there may be different regional alveolar pressures if airway obstruction differs between lung units, causing *pendel-luft* during the occlusion of the shutter.

Body plethysmography

This method can be considered a "gold standard", but requires complicated and bulky equipment.[2] The patient sits in a closed box, the "body plethysmograph", and breathes through a flowmeter that is open to the air within the box (see Fig 14.5). Respiratory flow is measured together with mouth and box pressure. This last pressure varies during breathing in inverse proportion to the variation in alveolar pressure, and is the effect of alveolar pressure causing mouth (and box) pressure to create airflow in and out of the lung. The gas in the box is then compressed and decompressed during inspiration and expiration, until pressure equilibrates between the alveoli and the box at the end of the breath. The trick is to convert the box signal to alveolar pressure. This can be done by closing the mouthpiece, asking the patient to breathe against the occluded airway. Mouth pressure will now be the same as alveolar pressure, because there is essentially no airflow in the airways. The mouth (and alveolar) pressure can then be compared with the simultaneously recorded box pressure to obtain a calibration or conversion factor. It may look simple at a glance, but there are a number of factors to take into account: first, there must be no fluttering of the subject's chin during the measurements, because this acts as a dampening capacitor, reducing the signal amplitude; second, gas temperature must not vary, because it would affect gas volumes and pressures in the lung and the box. Re-breathing conditioned air to and from a bag in the plethysmograph is one possibility for reducing temperature variations; a panting manoeuvre using small breaths to reduce heat loss is another.

Lung resistance

Lung resistance is the sum of airway and lung tissue resistances. The driving force is pleural pressure minus mouth pressure (transpulmonary pressure, Ptp), but this pressure difference is also used for expansion of the lung. Thus, the resistive pressure component must be separated from the elastic component, which can be done if the static pressure–volume curve of the lung is known or assumed. If resistance is measured during quiet breathing, it is customary to link end inspiratory and end expiratory pressure–volume points by a straight line, and calculate resistive pressure as the difference in pressure between the straight line and the measured transpulmonary pressure at that lung volume (or part of the tidal volume)

(Fig 17.2). Alternatively, if flow is suddenly stopped, the resistive pressure component rapidly drops to zero. So, by measuring transpulmonary pressure and airflow during a deep inspiration or expiration, with a shutter opening and closing the airway for periods of one second, both a pressure–volume curve and a resistance–volume curve can be constructed.[3] If, finally, the airflow is regulated, resistance can be defined in terms of lung volume and airflow, both of which play a most important role in the resistance value (Fig 17.3).

To calculate the resistance of the lung tissue itself, airway resistance has to be subtracted from lung resistance. In the anaesthetised, paralysed, and sedated patient who is undergoing mechanical ventilation, another simplified approach can be used to separate airway resistance from that of the tissue. As the recording is mostly done together with the measurement of total respiratory resistance, the method is described later.

Chest wall resistance

Chest wall resistance can hardly be measured in the spontaneously breathing subject, except as part of the total respiratory resistance (see later). It is, however, accessible during mechanical ventilation, as is the possibility of measuring chest wall compliance. Here the driving pressure is pleural or oesophageal pressure minus atmospheric pressure (or body surface pressure, if it differs from atmospheric). Again, the pressure comprises both the elastic and the resistive components, and they have to be separated to calculate the resistance. As with the analysis of lung resistance, a pressure–volume curve of the chest wall can be measured, or assumed to be linear between volume end points. The remaining pressure at a given volume is the resistive pressure which, divided by flow, gives the chest wall resistance. A complicating factor is the relatively large oesophageal pressure excursions caused by the beating heart. These variations can be almost half the magnitude of the pressure variations induced by the tidal volume. As the pressure waves from the ventilator and the heart are on the whole not in phase, an averaging procedure over several breaths may eliminate the influence of the heart beats. The value of analysing chest wall resistance is still unknown.

Total respiratory resistance

Total respiratory resistance (Rtot) is the sum of airway (Raw), lung tissue (Rlung tis), and chest wall (Rw) resistances:

$$R\text{tot} = R\text{aw} + R\text{lung tis} + R\text{w}.$$

It can be assessed only in the relaxed patient (or volunteer), and needs only the recording of airway pressure and airflow. In analogy with the

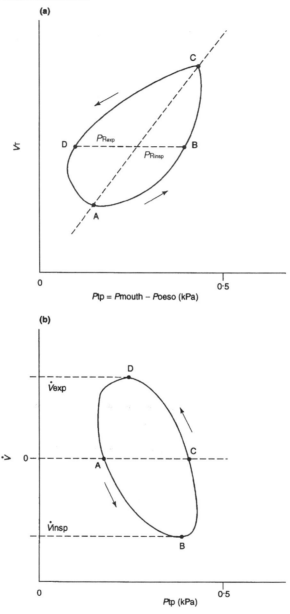

Fig 17.2 (a) Pressure–volume and (b) pressure–flow loops during a tidal breath. Assuming that the elastance is constant over the tidal volume, a straight line can be drawn between the maximum and minimum transpulmonary pressure (Ptp) on the pressure–volume loop. The difference in pressure between the loop and the straight line corresponds to the pressure needed to overcome resistive forces. These pressures (PRinsp, PRexp) can be divided by the simultaneously measured airflows (Vinsp, Vexp) to yield pulmonary resistance (airway and lung tissue resistance). Letters A, B, C, and D show simultaneous events in (a) and (b).

136

discussions above about the partitioning of elastic and resistive pressure components, the pressure–volume relationship of the total respiratory system has to be determined or assumed. This can be achieved by recording of a pressure–volume curve during breathing, or by interrupting inspiratory flow and measuring the sudden pressure drop that corresponds to the resistive pressure. This second measurement is easily achieved by setting a ventilator to deliver a constant inspiratory flow ("square wave") and

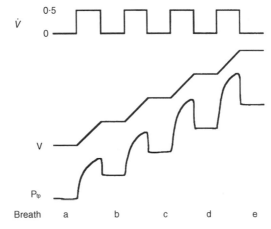

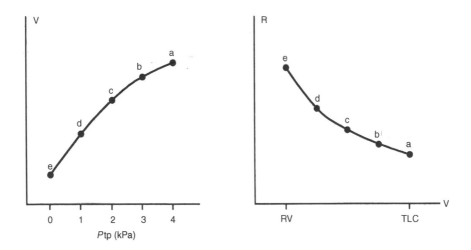

Fig 17.3   Shutter technique for the assessment of the pressure–volume curve of the lung and lung resistance over the vital capacity. By rapid airway occlusions and a flow regulator that maintains expiratory flow at a predetermined level, a volume–resistance curve can also be constructed. Note the increase in resistance with decreasing lung volume, an effect of the airway narrowing during expiration. Ptp, transpulmonary pressure.

applying an end inspiratory pause to give time for the pressure drop to be recorded before expiration begins.

The rapid end inspiratory occlusion of the airway can be used for a more detailed analysis of the resistance components if the end inspiratory pause is prolonged to at least two seconds.[4] The pressure drop at end inspiration is initially fast during the first few tenths of a second, but then slows down during the following one or two seconds, finally reaching a plateau. Although the causes of the rapid and slow phases are not fully clear, they are frequently assumed to reflect the airway resistive component (the initial rapid pressure drop) and the tissue component of both lung and chest wall (the slow pressure drop). This partitioning into an airway and a tissue component may not be correct and it is safer to refer to a "fast" and a "slow" component of the total resistance (compare Fig 16.3). Using this analysis, the increased total resistance that has been found in patients with acute respiratory distress syndrome (ARDS) has been shown to be caused by an increase in the slow "tissue" component more than in the fast "airway" component.[5] Moreover, the moderate increase in the fast component may be explained by a decrease in lung volume that is a regular finding in ARDS.[6]

There is another, completely different technique for assessing resistance. It is based on an oscillation of the lung and chest wall, by applying a loud speaker or oscillating pump to the airway. If the patient breathes air, airway pressure varies synchronously with the breathing. The superimposed oscillations by the loud speaker, or pump, will increase or decrease in magnitude as a consequence of resonance phenomena in the lung and chest wall, and they can be used to calculate the total resistance.[7] The influence of the different components of the total resistance will vary with the superimposed oscillating frequency, so, if the frequency is altered over a specific range, from about 3 to 10 hertz, a partitioning of the different resistance components can be made, at least in theory.

Inertia

The acceleration of air into the lungs and acceleration of the movement of the chest wall tissue, including the abdominal wall and abdominal organs, require additional force which adds to the power demand and the respiratory work. Normally, the pressure needed to bring about this acceleration of gas and tissue movement, that is, to overcome their inertia, is very small and in practice not measurable. It has therefore been neglected. When, however, gas and tissue are exposed to very high accelerations, the inertia may be sufficiently large to contribute significantly to the power needed and the work performed. A situation in which this may occur is high frequency breathing. Normally, this is executed by a ventilator. In yoga exercises, however, a breathing pattern is included that consists of rapid shallow breathing. Yogi can breathe at a rate of 4 breaths/ second for an hour or more.[8] The tidal volume is as large as 0·35 litre, resulting in a minute volume of about 90 litres. With this breathing pattern, work of acceleration contributed 25–30% to the total resistive work. (Severe hypocapnia may have been expected, but the Pa_{CO_2} was within the normal range, with a mean of 4·8 kPa (36 mm Hg).) This was a consequence of the reduced tidal volume and high respiratory work, with an increase of O_2 uptake to 800 ml/min. This corresponds to the work needed during moderate exercise on an ergometer cycle (60–70 watts).

Another condition in which inertia during breathing may be appreciable is ventilation with a heavy gas or a fluid. Liquids based on perfluorocarbons are being tried in the ventilation of animals with acute respiratory failure, and there have been a few trials in newborn children with severe respiratory distress.[9] This fluid has a specific weight of 1·8, and may exert inertia during ventilation. The work to overcome it has to be done by the ventilator and should not be a burden to the patient.

Power and work of breathing

As mentioned earlier, the product of pressure and flow is power. It is important for the ventilator manufacturer to know this, so that the machine is designed to deliver enough power even in situations of severe airway obstruction or lung stiffness. (Damage of the lungs by high pressure, or volume, is another story, but will set limits on the practical use of mechanical ventilation.)

The respiratory work is the integral over time of power, or the product of pressure and volume. It can be expressed as work per breath or, more reasonably, per minute. Only resistive pulmonary work can be measured in the spontaneously breathing patient. The reason is that the pressure–volume curve of the chest wall is not known, and can hardly be measured.[10] This makes it impossible to define the total pressure and work generated by the respiratory muscles. The resistive work, on the other hand, requires knowledge of the pressure generated to produce airflow, and it can be determined as described previously. Although both pulmonary resistive power and work are of definite importance in determining respiratory muscle performance and work, they are seldom measured. This may be an area of future scientific interest, together with metabolic studies of the muscles. It was demonstrated some 20 years ago that acute exacerbations of patients with severe chronic bronchitis caused a complete depletion of the energy rich substrates, both in intercostal muscles and in quadriceps femoris.[11] The depletion in the thigh muscle was comparable to that seen in athletes after maximum leg exercise!

In the ventilator treated patient, total respiratory work can be determined as the product of airway pressure and volume. As for the spontaneously breathing subject, it is seldom used. It might prove able to predict when a patient is apt to manage breathing on his or her own.

1 Jackson AC, Milhorn HT Jr, Norman JR. A reevaluation of the interrupter technique for airway resistance measurement. *J Appl Physiol* 1974;**36**:264–8.
2 DuBois AB, Botelho SY, Comroe JH Jr. A new method for measuring airway resistance in man using a body plethysmograph: Values in normal subjects and in patients with respiratory disease. *J Clin Invest* 1956;**35**:327–35.
3 Jonson B. A method for determination of pulmonary elastic recoil and resistance at a regulated flow rate. *Scand J Clin Lab Invest* 1969;**24**:115–25.
4 Broseghini C, Brandolese R, Poggi R, Polese G, Manzin E, Milic-Emili J, Rossi A. Respiratory mechanics during the first day of mechanical ventilation in patients with pulmonary edema and chronic airway obstruction. *Am Rev Respir Dis* 1988;**138**:355–61.
5 Tantucci C, Corbeil C, Chasse M, Braidy J, Matar N, Milic-Emili J. Flow resistance in patients with chronic obstructive pulmonary disease in acute respiratory failure. Effects of flow and volume. *Am Rev Respir Dis* 1991;**144**:384–9.
6 Pelosi P, Cereda M, Foti G, Giacomini M, Pesenti A. Alterations of lung and chest wall mechanics in patients with acute lung injury: effects of positive end-expiratory pressure. *Am J Respir Crit Care Med* 1995;**152**:531–7.
7 Aronsson H, Solymar L, Dempsey J, Bjure J, Olsson T, Bake B. A modified forced oscillation technique for measurements of respiratory resistance. *J Appl Physiol* 1977;**42**:650–5.
8 Frostell C, Pande J, Hedenstierna G. Effects of high frequency breathing on pulmonary ventilation and gas exchange. *J Appl Physiol* 1983;**55**:1374–8.
9 Tütüncü AS, Faithfull NS, Lachmann B. Comparison of ventilatory support with intratracheal perfluororocarbon administration and conventional mechanical ventilation in animals with acute respiratory failure. *Am Rev Respir Dis* 1993;**148**:785–92.
10 Jonson B, Olsson GB. Measurement of the work of breathing to overcome pulmonary viscous resistance. *Scand J Clin Lab Invest* 1971;**28**:135–40.
11 Gertz I, Hedenstierna G, Hellers G, Wahren J. Muscle metabolism in patient with chronic obstructive lung disease and acute respiratory failure. *Clin Sci Mol Med* 1977;**52**:395–403.

18: Gas exchange: hypoventilation and gas diffusion

General

The oxygenation of blood and the elimination of CO_2 from the blood can be assessed by a blood gas analysis. It gives the ultimate result of the gas exchanging capacity of the lung. As stated in Part I, impaired gas exchange, causing hypoxaemia and hypercapnia, can be caused by: (1) hypoventilation, (2) diffusion impairment, (3) ventilation–perfusion mismatch, and (4) right-to-left shunt. If any of these impairments exist, the Pao_2 and $Paco_2$ values seldom indicate what is wrong, unless arterial blood samples are taken under different experimental conditions (see Table 8.1). There might even be an abnormality in spite of normal blood gases. Compensatory mechanisms or other simultaneously occurring abnormalities may balance the effect of the primary disturbance. One example is the asthmatic patient, who may have a normal Pao_2 despite a ventilation–perfusion ($\dot{V}_A/\dot{Q}$) mismatch. The explanation is that the asthmatic patient often has a high cardiac output because of medication with sympathomimetic drugs, and the hyperkinetic circulation allows a higher than normal venous Po_2. This facilitates the oxygenation of blood and reduces the desaturating effect of blood that is passing through regions with low $\dot{V}_A/\dot{Q}$ ratios.

To find the cause of impaired gas exchange, or to reveal a more subtle disturbance that may not lower Pao_2, something more than blood gas analysis is needed. In this chapter different causes of disturbances and methods for their disclosure are discussed. The technical aspects of blood gas analysis are not dealt with here. The interested reader is referred to Peter Driscoll et al: *A Simple Guide to Blood Gas Analysis* (BMJ Publishing Group 1997).

Hypoventilation

The commonly used definition of hypoventilation is hypercapnia or CO_2 retention, rather than a threshold value of minute or alveolar ventilation. In a hypermetabolic state, caused by exercise, fever, or even heavy loading of CO_2 stores by intravenous feeding, minute ventilation can be high, and

141

$P\text{CO}_2$ may also be elevated. Large dead space ventilation in obstructive lung disease and pulmonary embolism increases the ventilatory demand. In addition, $\dot{V}\text{A}/\dot{Q}$ mismatch and, in particular, large shunts let the mixed venous blood pass through the lungs with impeded or no release of CO_2. The blood from these "low" $\dot{V}\text{A}/\dot{Q}$ and shunt regions elevates the $P\text{aCO}_2$. Thus, high $P\text{aCO}_2$ values may not indicate a low minute ventilation, but that it is insufficient under the prevailing conditions.

Hypoventilation also lowers the $P\text{aO}_2$ in approximate proportion to the increase in $P\text{aCO}_2$ (or more), as can be seen from the alveolar gas equation (see box). This means that hypoxaemia can be seen in patients breathing air, but the effect on $P\text{aO}_2$ during ventilation with oxygen enriched gas is

---

Alveolar gas equations

Alveolar oxygen tension ($P\text{AO}_2$)

$$P\text{AO}_2 = P\text{IO}_2 - \frac{P\text{ACO}_2}{R} + \left[P\text{ACO}_2 \times F\text{IO}_2 \times \frac{1-R}{R} \right]$$

where $P\text{IO}_2$ = inspired oxygen tension; $P\text{ACO}_2$ = alveolar CO_2 tension (assumed to equal arterial $P\text{CO}_2$); R = respiratory exchange ratio (normally in the range of $0\cdot8$–$1\cdot0$); $F\text{IO}_2$ = inspired oxygen fraction.

The term within brackets compensates for the larger O_2 uptake than CO_2 elimination over the alveolar–capillary membranes.

A simplified equation can be written without the compensation term:

$$P\text{AO}_2 = P\text{IO}_2 - \frac{P\text{ACO}_2}{R}.$$

Alveolar ventilation

The alveolar ventilation ($\dot{V}\text{A}$) can be expressed:

$$\dot{V}\text{A} = f \times (V\text{T} - V\text{D})$$

where f = breaths/min; $V\text{T}$ = tidal volume and $V\text{D}$ = physiological dead space.

The alveolar ventilation can also be derived from:

$$\dot{V}\text{CO}_2 = c \times \dot{V}\text{A} \times F\text{ACO}_2$$

where $\dot{V}\text{CO}_2$ = CO_2 elimination/min; c = conversion constant; $F\text{ACO}_2$ = alveolar CO_2 concentration.

If $\dot{V}\text{A}$ is expressed in l/min, $\dot{V}\text{CO}_2$ in ml/min and $F\text{ACO}_2$ is replaced by $P\text{ACO}_2$ in mm Hg, $c = 0\cdot863$. By rearranging:

$$\dot{V}\text{A} = \frac{\dot{V}\text{CO}_2 \times 0\cdot863}{P\text{ACO}_2}.$$

hardly noticeable. An increase in Pa_{CO_2} from 5·32 to 10·64 kPa (40 to 80 mm Hg) lowers Pa_{O_2} to around 6·65 kPa (50 mm Hg) during air breathing. During ventilation with 50% O_2, the ideal Pa_{O_2} is about 39·9 kPa (300 mm Hg), but the normal range is larger than during air breathing, so that a fall in Pa_{O_2} to 33·25 kPa (250 mm Hg), caused by hypercapnia, would not be considered a sign of any important dysfunction. Moreover, any fall in Pa_{O_2} can easily be corrected by elevation of the inspired O_2 concentration.

The detection of hypoventilation is thus based on a blood gas analysis. Detection of the underlying cause requires evaluation of: (1) minute ventilation, (2) dead space, (3) whole body CO_2 production, and (4) shunt. Ventilation–perfusion mismatch contributes to only a small degree and can be neglected in most situations.

Diffusion in the gas phase

Airflow in the airways is convectional down to the respiratory bronchioles. The very last stage of gas transport is considered to be by diffusion, which is an effect of the rapid increase in overall airway and alveolar diameter, making bulk flow (convection) very low. Diffusion, in the presence of a concentration gradient within the airway and alveolus, then becomes more important than convection.

The diffusion rate in the gas phase has been studied to increase understanding of basic physiology, but it is not part of any clinical investigation of a patient. Its importance still remains unclear, although there is general acceptance that, in the presence of enlarged airspaces, as in emphysema, a considerable O_2 and CO_2 gradient may exist within the alveoli.[1]

The way to demonstrate the presence of stratification of a gas in the gas exchanging unit has been by comparison of the slope of expired gases of different weights. The heavier the gas, the less it is able to diffuse. Thus, if a heavy gas displays a steeper alveolar plateau than a lighter gas, this could indicate that the heavy gas has not mixed to the same extent as the lighter one.[1] The problem is that the gases may also have different solubilities in blood and lung tissue, and have different viscosities which, together with their different densities, influence the resistance to convectional gas flow. All these factors make the quantification of diffusion limitation in the gas phase difficult to study. If a small lung unit could be studied separately, many of the confounding factors could be eliminated or their influence reduced. This is something that an anaesthetist could work on.

Diffusion across the alveolar–capillary membranes

Another aspect of diffusion is that across the alveolar–capillary membranes. It may play a more important role in limiting oxygenation of blood

143

than stratification of gas within the airway and alveolus. It has been studied by many research groups and is the subject of many clinical investigations.

The test of the diffusion capacity of the lung is frequently called the "transfer test" to clarify that the test is dependent not only on membrane characteristics, but also on other factors such as lung area available for diffusion and capillary blood volume. This should be remembered when interpreting the results.

The diffusion capacity can be quantified by a gas that is limited by its diffusion across the alveolar–capillary membranes and not by the pulmonary blood flow. No gas can meet these criteria to the full extent, but carbon monoxide (CO) comes close. Its diffusion through the membranes is slightly slower than for O_2, by a factor of 1·34, and its avid binding to haemoglobin makes the rate of blood flow only a modestly limiting factor. The partial pressure of CO built up during the test at the low CO concentrations used (usually 0·3% in inspired gas during a single breath test) causes a minor counterpressure in the blood, which can be disregarded when calculating the diffusion capacity in most situations. Heavy smokers may, however, have an arterial CO tension (Paco) of 0·67–1·33 kPa (5–10 mm Hg). In these cases Paco must be taken into consideration to yield accurate results. Another gas that has been tested is nitric oxide (NO), which is even more soluble in blood than CO. When, however, it was learned in the late 1980s that NO is a most powerful vasodilator, including of the pulmonary vascular tree, it became evident that NO was not suitable. It could increase the pulmonary capillary blood volume and so affect the transfer factor under study.

The CO transfer test is simply a maximum expiration, followed by a maximum inspiration of a low concentration of CO (about 0·3%) and helium in air, a breath-hold to allow CO, but not the poorly soluble helium, to diffuse to the capillary blood, and an expiration so that a sample of alveolar gas can be collected for CO and helium determination. The uptake of CO can then be calculated and be divided by the alveolar CO tension, to give the transfer factor. For further details, see Fig 18.1 and the box. Helium gas is inhaled to correct for dilution of the inspired CO by the remaining air in the lung, corresponding to the residual volume (RV).[2] It also enables calculation of the diffusion capacity per litre of the functional residual capacity (FRC). Lung volume is one of the determinants of the transfer factor, so by taking the FRC into account the influence of other factors on the diffusion rate may become more discernible. Also, as diffusion starts as soon as the gas has entered the alveoli and continues as long as CO is in the lung, a correct diffusion time must be calculated. This is taken as the time between when 30% of the vital capacity (VC) has been inspired and the start of the collection of the expired gas sample, normally 1 litre after the start of expiration. The first expired litre is discarded because it also contains dead space gas. If the test is done in a patient with a VC of less than 2 litres, or close to it, however, the test has to be modified, by either discarding less gas before sample collection or reducing the gas sample. The second may be preferable, because it will increase the likelihood that the dead space has been washed out before gas collection. The reason that as much as a litre of gas, if possible, is collected is that there is a change in the CO concentration during the expiration, so that a single point on the expired volume curve is less representative. This variation is an effect of different Va/V and Va/Q ratios, which cause varying dilutions of the inspired gas and its uptake, as well as varying diffusion rates in the presence of fibrotic disease. The regional differences in alveolar CO concentrations provide the reason why it is desirable that the patient expire at a moderate expiratory flow which enables simultaneous emptying of all or most lung units.

The diffusion capacity for CO is normally in the range of 100–150 ml/min per mm Hg.[3] As can be expected, it is reduced in fibrotic disease with thickened alveolar–capillary membranes. It is also reduced in alveolar oedema and proteinosis, and when capillary blood volume is reduced as in pulmonary hypotension and emphysema.[4] In emphysema, the expanded alveoli compress the capillary bed and reduce the blood volume. There is a marked decrease in the diffusion capacity in emphysema, despite the alveolar–capillary membranes being normal or even thinner than normal.

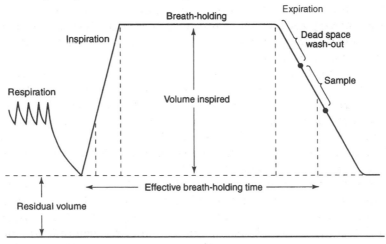

Fig 18.1 Procedures for the single breath CO transfer test (diffusion capacity): (1) a maximum expiration to RV; (2) full inspiration to TLC in less than 4 seconds; (3) gas inspired is CO (about 0·3%), He (5–10%), O_2 (21%) in N_2; (4) the breath is held for 8 seconds; (5) full expiration to RV at a flow rate of about 0·5 l/s; (6) after the expiration of 0·7–1·0 litre, collection of 0·6–0·9 litre gas sample for analysis of CO and He concentrations; (7) breath-hold time is calculated from one third of inspired VC to when half of the expired gas sample has been taken. Further details on equations are given in Table 18.2.

145

In analogy with the effect of reduced capillary blood volume, anaemia also lowers the diffusion capacity. Polycythaemia, on the other hand, increases the diffusion rate. Chronic bronchitis or asthma interferes only to a minor extent with the diffusion capacity. A minor decrease can be expected on the grounds of uneven distribution of the inspired gas, but it will hardly cause a pathological value. In the event of a clear decrease in the diffusion capacity in chronic bronchitis, it is more likely that the patient has smoked and has a high $P_{A}CO$. This can be calculated from the spectrophotometric determination of carboxyhaemoglobin (COHb) and entered into the equation in the box.

As the capillary blood volume has a considerable impact on the diffusion capacity, as measured, it would be advantageous if its effect on the diffusion value could be separated from the other causes of diffusion limitation. This is indeed possible by repeating the test at two different inspired O_2 concentrations. The rationale is that O_2 and CO compete for the binding

---

Equations for CO transfer test

The flow of a gas ($\dot{V}_{gas}$) across the alveolar–capillary membranes can be written:

$$\dot{V}_{gas} = \frac{A}{T} \times D(P_A - P_C)$$

where A = surface area available for gas flow, T = membrane thickness, and D approximates solubility of gas in the tissue divided by the square of the molecular weight of the gas, P_A and P_C = alveolar and capillary gas tension, respectively.

In practice T and A cannot be measured, only an overall transfer (or diffusion) factor, T_L (D_L):

$$T_L \text{ (or } D_L) = A/T \times D$$

$$V_{gas} = T_L \times (P_A - P_C).$$

Using CO as test gas and assuming $P_C = 0$, the equation can be rarranged:

$$T_LCO = \dot{V}CO/P_ACO.$$

The inspired CO will be diluted by the remaining air in the lung at RV. This can be taken into account if a poorly soluble, "non-diffusible" gas is inhaled simultaneously with CO. That is why helium is used during the assessment of T_LCO. Then:

$$T_LCO = b \times V_A/t \times \log_{10}[(F_ICO \times F_AHe)/(F_ACO \times F_IHe)]$$

where b = dimensional constant (53·6 if SI units are used; 160 if conventional units are used), V_A = alveolar volume (can be deducted from the dilution of the inspired He), t = breath-hold time (seconds), F_A = alveolar concentrations of CO and He, and F_I = inspired concentrations of CO and He.

---

sites in the haemoglobin molecule.[5] Thus, if inspired O_2 is increased, more O_2 will bind to the haemoglobin, and less CO. This enables a calculation of both the "membrane" factor (Dm) and the capillary blood volume component (Dc). There is an inverse relationship between the overall diffusion capacity of the lung (D_{LCO}), and its two components:

$$1/D_{LCO} = [1/Dm] + [1/Dc].$$

The diffusion capacity can also be measured during steady state re-breathing of CO. The steady state technique is virtually independent of the gas distribution, but as this is also mostly a minor problem with the single breath technique, it may not be sufficient to encourage the use of the steady state technique. If a VC manoeuvre cannot be performed, then the steady state technique may offer an advantage. There is also a technique based on the breathing of oxygen at different concentrations. It can be claimed to be the method for measuring diffusion of a gas of more clinical interest. Oxygen diffusion capacity can, however, be calculated from the CO diffusion with good accuracy, leaving little to inspire the use of the O_2 technique. Neither technique is frequently used any longer, because they are more demanding.

The application of a transfer test to anaesthetised or ventilator treated patients has not been extensive. This is surprising, because it should be easy to execute in a standardised manner and it may offer information that is not easily retrieved from other measurements.[6] An increased appearance in the intensive care setting might be anticipated!

1 Scheid P, Piiper J. Intrapulmonary gas mixing and stratification. In: West JB, ed. *Pulmonary gas exchange*, vol 1. New York: Academic Press, 1980: 87–130.
2 Cotes JE, Chinn DJ, Quanjer PH, Roca J, Yernault JC. Standardization of the measurement of transfer factor (Diffusing Capacity). *Eur Respir J Suppl* 1993;**16**:41–52.
3 Knudson RJ, Kaltenborn WT, Knudson DE, Burrows B. The single-breath carbon monoxide diffusing capacity. Reference equations derived from a healthy nonsmoking population and effects of hematocrit. *Am Rev Respir Dis* 1987;**135**:805–11.
4 Morrison NJ, Abboud RT, Ramadan F, Miller RR, Gibson NN, Evans KG, et al. Comparison of single breath carbon monoxide diffusing capacity and pressure-volume curves in detecting emphysema. *Am Rev Respir Dis* 1989;**139**:1179–87.
5 Roughton FJW, Forster RE. Relative importance of diffusion and chemical reaction rates in determining rate of exchange of gases in the human lung, with special references to true diffusing capacity of pulmonary membrane and volume of blood in the lung capillaries. *J Appl Physiol* 1957;**11**:290–302.
6 Macnaughton PD, Evans TW. Measurement of lung volume and D_{LCO} in acute respiratory failure. *Am J Respir Crit Care Med* 1994;**150**:770–5.

19:   Gas exchange: ventilation–perfusion relationships and shunt

General

The most common cause of hypoxaemia is ventilation–perfusion ($\dot{V}A/\dot{Q}$) mismatch. It occurs essentially in all patients with obstructive lung disease and in most patients with restrictive or fibrotic lung disease, which is less appreciated. Moreover, a $\dot{V}A/\dot{Q}$ disturbance will affect the CO_2 elimination and increase $Paco_2$, contrary to most expectations. It is often mistakenly said that the CO_2–haemoglobin dissociation curve is linear in the physiological range, so that hyperventilating areas of the lung compensate for the hypoventilating ones. Theoretical calculations show that CO_2 retention can be more marked than O_2 desaturation in the presence of $\dot{V}A/\dot{Q}$ mismatch. That this has been overlooked is presumably because hypoxaemia stimulates increased ventilation, which returns the $Paco_2$ to normal or near normal. Pao_2, on the other hand, cannot be corrected any more by increased ventilation, because the normally ventilated regions are able to oxygenate the blood almost fully (haemoglobin saturation of around 98%), and a further increase in their ventilation does not raise the saturation much further. Thus, 100% saturation of blood is not reached until the alveolar, and arterial, Po_2 are almost 26·7 kPa (200 mm Hg).

There are several approaches to disclosing $\dot{V}A/\dot{Q}$ mismatch, ranging from a single compartment analysis, over a three compartment reconstruction, to complex multicompartment models. They are discussed in this chapter.

Single compartment analysis

For a given $\dot{V}A/\dot{Q}$ ratio of the lungs, there is a pair of Pao_2 and $Paco_2$ values that matches the $\dot{V}A/\dot{Q}$ ratio for a given inspired O_2 concentration. It has also to be assumed that there is no diffusion impairment. This relationship is given in the Fenn and Rahn diagram (Fig 19.1). It can be seen that, in a situation in which there is ventilation but no blood flow ($\dot{V}A/\dot{Q}$ ratio of infinity, that is, dead space), Pao_2 equals Pio_2 and $Paco_2$ is zero

148

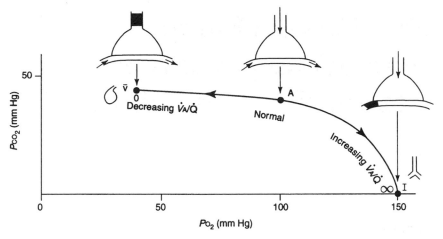

Fig 19.1 Oxygen–carbon dioxide diagram showing the effect of different ventilation-perfusion ratios ($\dot{V}_A/\dot{Q}$ line). Three lung units are shown: shunt (located at the mixed venous point v̄), normal (ideal) ventilation–perfusion ratio (A), dead space (located at the inspired gas point I). (Reprinted from West,[1] with permission.)

(if there was any blood flow). At the other end of the possible range, there is blood flow but no ventilation ($\dot{V}_A/\dot{Q}$ ratio of zero, that is, shunt) with P_{AO_2} equalling $P\bar{v}_{O_2}$ and P_{ACO_2} being similar to $P\bar{v}_{CO_2}$. In between, unique pairs of P_{AO_2} and P_{ACO_2} values match all possible $\dot{V}_A/\dot{Q}$ ratios. Thus, a blood gas can tell you the average $\dot{V}_A/\dot{Q}$ ratio of that lung, assuming no diffusion impairment. It may be argued whether this is useful information, but it is presented here to help understand the relationships between blood gases and $\dot{V}_A/\dot{Q}$ ratio.

Three compartment analysis

A more advanced, but still simple, modelling of the $\dot{V}_A/\dot{Q}$ distribution is the three compartment analysis where one compartment is ventilated but non-perfused (dead space), one is ventilated and perfused (ideal compartment), and one is perfused but not ventilated (shunt) (Fig 19.2). In the context of gas exchange, it is the physiological dead space, that is, the sum of anatomical and alveolar dead spaces, that is of interest. The single breath N_2 wash-out, although suitable for assessing anatomical dead space, is not suitable for measurement of physiological dead space (see chapter 15). The physiological dead space can be calculated according to the Bohr formula, which is presented in the box. As can be seen, it requires the collection of a representative alveolar gas sample. This is difficult because there is no single alveolar CO_2 concentration, but a range of values. Also, the end tidal CO_2 concentration that can be measured by a fast responding instrument, for example, an infrared meter, is not identical to the mean alveolar CO_2

149

concentration. The alveolar sample can be replaced by the arterial CO_2 concentration (or tension), as proposed by Enghoff[2] which results in the familiar equation:

$$V_D/V_T = (P_{ACO_2} - P_{\bar{E}CO_2})/P_{ACO_2}$$

where V_D is dead space, V_T is tidal volume, P_{ACO_2} is arterial P_{CO_2}, $P_{\bar{E}CO_2}$ is mixed expired CO_2 tension. The derivation of the equation is shown in the box.

The $P_{\bar{E}CO_2}$ can be measured by collecting the expired gas in a bag, shaking it to ensure thorough mixing, and then measuring the concentration or partial pressure by a gas absorption technique or infrared spectroscopy. The infrared meter also enables continuous, on line recording of expired gas, and by multiplying instantaneous P_{CO_2} with the con-

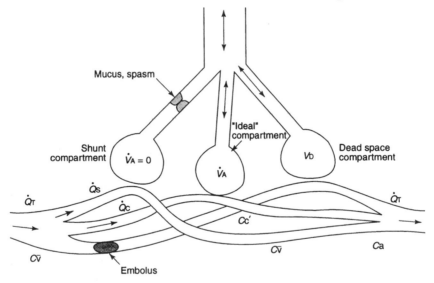

Fig 19.2   A three compartment analysis of gas exchange. One compartment is ventilated but not perfused (dead space), one is ventilated and perfused (the ideal compartment), and one is perfused but not ventilated (shunt). In practice, however, there is no sharp distinction between compartments. There are units that are ventilated in excess of their perfusion and they will be incorporated in both the dead space compartment and the ideal one. There are other units that are perfused in excess of their ventilation and they will be located in both the shunt compartment and the ideal one. The distinction between the compartments will depend on the solubility of the tracer gases that are used. The use of O_2 for the assessment of shunt will not enable calculation of "true shunt" but will also include regions with "low" $V_A/\dot{Q}$ regions. The "oxygen shunt" might be better described as venous admixture (see also Fig 10.3). By the same token, dead space, as assessed by standard CO_2 elimination techniques, will include regions with high $V_A/\dot{Q}$ ratios. Finally, the "ideal" compartment will include regions with $V_A/\dot{Q}$ ratios ranging from low to high and not only compartments with a $V_A/\dot{Q}$ ratio of 1·0.

Derivation of the physiological dead space equation

$$F\dot{E} \times V_T = F_A(V_T - V_D) + (F_I \times V_D) \qquad (1)$$

By rearranging:

$$\frac{V_D}{V_T} = \frac{F_A - F\dot{E}}{F_A - F_I} \qquad (2)$$

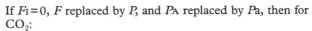

If $F_I = 0$, F replaced by P, and P_A replaced by P_a, then for CO_2:

$$\frac{V_D}{V_T} = \frac{Pa_{CO_2} - P\bar{E}_{CO_2}}{Pa_{CO_2}} \qquad (3)$$

where $F\dot{E}$, F_A, F_I are mixed expired, alveolar, inspired gas concentrations respectively, and V_T, V_D, and V_A are tidal volume, dead space, and part of the tidal volume to perfused alveoli respectively.

tinuously measured expired gas flow, and integrating the signal over time, $P\bar{E}_{CO_2}$ is obtained.

The end tidal P_{CO_2} ($P_{ET_{CO_2}}$) was the value that Bohr initially proposed as a measure of Pa_{CO_2}. There is, however, a difference between them, which can be appreciated when looking at an expiratory CO_2 curve. It shows a sloping alveolar plateau, indicating that alveolar gas that has not been expired contains a higher concentration of CO_2 than gas that has been expired (compare Fig 15.4). Although in healthy people this difference between Pa_{CO_2} and $P_{ET_{CO_2}}$ is no larger than 266–400 Pa (2–3 mm Hg), it increases in lung disease. Also, during anaesthesia the difference in Pa and P_{ET} for CO_2 is increased to, on average, 1·06 kPa (8 mm Hg).[3]

A difficulty with this analysis is that the solubility of CO_2 in blood is such that lung units with high $V_A/\dot{Q}$ ratios also contribute to the calculated dead space. To enable a more distinct separation of dead space from ventilated and perfused units, a gas with higher solubility than CO_2 must be used. Thus, the dead space value will depend on the tracer gas. The great use of CO_2 is because it has a fairly high solubility and is always available in the expired gas.

Shunt can be assessed from the oxygenation of blood and is determined by an equation that is identical in design to that of dead space:[4]

$$\dot{Q}s/\dot{Q}t = (Cc'_{O_2} - Ca_{O_2})/(Cc'_{O_2} - C\bar{v}_{O_2})$$

where $\dot{Q}t$ is cardiac output, $\dot{Q}c$ is blood flow through ventilated lung tissue, $\dot{Q}s$ is shunt, and Ca, Cc', and $C\bar{v}$ are concentrations (of O_2) in arterial, end capillary, and mixed venous blood, respectively. The derivation of the equation is shown in the box.

151

Derivation of the venous admixture ("shunt") equation

$$Ca \times \dot{Q}t = (Cc' \times \dot{Q}c) + (C\bar{v} \times \dot{Q}s) \qquad (1)$$

$$\dot{Q}c = \dot{Q}t - \dot{Q}s \qquad (2)$$

Inserting eqn (2) into eqn (1):

$$Ca \times \dot{Q}t = Cc \times (\dot{Q}t - \dot{Q}s) + C\bar{v} \times \dot{Q}s$$

Rearranging:

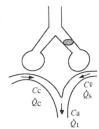

$$\frac{\dot{Q}s}{\dot{Q}t} = \frac{Cc' - Ca}{Cc' - C\bar{v}}$$

where Cc', Ca, $C\bar{v}$ = oxygen content in pulmonary end-capillary, arterial, and mixed venous blood, respectively. $\dot{Q}t$ = cardiac output; $\dot{Q}c$ = capillary flow and $\dot{Q}s$ = shunt.

As for the discussion on dead space, the shunt, as assessed by the O_2 technique, includes regions with low $\dot{V}A/\dot{Q}$ ratios. To separate shunt from lung units with any ventilation (and blood flow), a gas with an extremely low solubility in blood has to be used. Thus, the "oxygen shunt" is not a pure shunt and should preferably be called "venous admixture". This term denotes a blood flow that contributes to the desaturation of arterial blood (compare Fig 10.3).

There is a trick to separating the shunt from regions with low $\dot{V}A/\dot{Q}$ ratios. This is to calculate the shunt during pure O_2 breathing, which eliminates any contribution to the shunt value from regions with low $\dot{V}A/\dot{Q}$ ratios. This analysis often, however, yields contradictory results and interference with the measured variable has also been noticed, such as absorption collapse (atelectasis) and increased shunt as a result of inhibition of hypoxic pulmonary vasoconstriction.

As the O_2 method has limitations, as described above, attempts have been made to find techniques that give a better description of the shunt. This can be achieved by infusing a gas of very low solubility in blood so that, when it passes through the lung capillaries, it is retained only in those regions that are perfused but not ventilated. In gas filled lung units, even if ventilation is poor, the low solubility of the tracer gas causes its diffusion to the alveoli and its subsequent elimination via the airways. Xenon is a gas with relatively low solubility in blood (blood:gas partition coefficient, $\lambda = 0.19$). By collecting an arterial and a mixed venous blood sample, the retention (R) can be calculated as $Ca/C\bar{v}$, where Ca and $C\bar{v}$ are arterial and mixed venous tracer gas concentrations. The equation:

$$R = Ca/C\bar{v} = \lambda/(\lambda + \dot{V}A/\dot{Q})$$

gives the relationship between the retention of the tracer gas, the blood gas partition coefficient, and the $\dot{V}_A/\dot{Q}$ for an "inert" gas (that is, chemically inactive in blood). It can be seen that a λ of 0·19 (xenon) and a normal $\dot{V}_A/\dot{Q}$ ratio of 1·0 gives an R of 16%. For O_2 the situation is more complex because the gas is not "inert" but combines with haemoglobin according to the O_2 dissociation curve. However, If a single value for λ (O_2) of 0·9 is used, to enable a simplified comparison with the xenon retention, and a $\dot{V}_A/\dot{Q}$ ratio of 1, the corresponding R is about 50%. For a lung unit with a lower $\dot{V}_A/\dot{Q}$ ratio, more of the gas is retained. Thus, there is at least a threefold difference in the degree of retention in normal $\dot{V}_A/\dot{Q}$ units for these two gases. It is obvious that xenon is the better gas for discriminating true shunt. By infusing radioactive xenon (^{133}Xe) intravenously, the shunt can be detected by external detectors, positioned over the chest.[5]

Although xenon is a better gas for assessing true shunt than O_2, it is still not ideal, some gas being retained also in normal $\dot{V}_A/\dot{Q}$ units. Sulphur hexafluoride (SF_6) has extremely low solubility in blood ($\lambda = 0·006$), and is therefore almost completely eliminated from the capillary blood in lung units with normal $\dot{V}_A/\dot{Q}$ ratios, and to a major extent in lung regions with $\dot{V}_A/\dot{Q}$ ratios as low as 0·005–0·010, as can be calculated by entering SF_6 into the equation. As a result of its extremely low solubility, intravenous infusion of SF_6 can also be used for assessing individual lung blood flow, if expired gas can be collected via a double lumen endobronchial catheter. This is because differences in the $\dot{V}_A/\dot{Q}$ ratio and the venous/arterial tracer gas concentration ratio of each lung will have minimal impact on the elimination of SF_6 gas. By this means it compares favourably with CO_2 and xenon elimination, which have been used more frequently for such purposes.[6]

Despite their theoretical advantages, neither xenon nor SF_6 has been extensively used for assessing true shunt (or individual lung blood flow), mainly because of the difficulties in handling gases of low solubility and the need for sophisticated equipment for analysis (for example, mass spectrometer or gas chromatograph). Sulphur hexafluoride is, however, used, together with other gases of different solubilities in blood, for the assessment of the $\dot{V}_A/\dot{Q}$ distribution.

Multicompartment analysis

By using more than one or two gases with different solubilities in blood, a more detailed analysis of $\dot{V}_A/\dot{Q}$ can be made. Thus, Wagner and co-workers[7 8] have developed a multiple inert gas elimination technique (MIGET) which is based on the retention and elimination of several (in practice six) "inert" gases (gases obeying Henry's law, that is, showing a linear relationship between partial pressure and concentration in blood, such as SF_6 and xenon) with different solubilities in blood. The retention

(a)

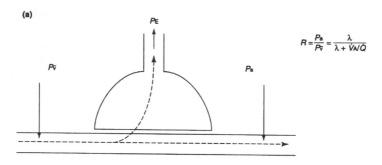

$$R = \frac{P_a}{P_{\bar{v}}} = \frac{\lambda}{\lambda + \dot{V}_A/\dot{Q}}$$

(b)

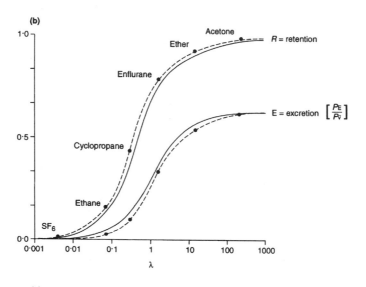

(c)

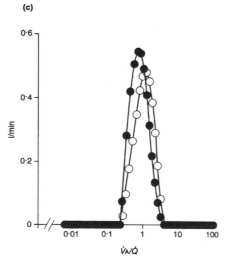

154

and excretion values for the six gases can be used to allocate ventilation and blood flow to a number of hypothetical compartments (for example, 50) ranging from shunt ($\dot{V}_A/\dot{Q}=0$) over compartments with low, normal, and high $\dot{V}_A/\dot{Q}$ ratios to dead space ($\dot{V}_A/\dot{Q}=\infty$). A schematic drawing of the basic principles is shown in Fig 19.3 and some examples of $\dot{V}_A/\dot{Q}$ disturbance in Fig 19.4. The fundamental equations that enable the calculation of $\dot{V}_A/\dot{Q}$ are deducted from two basic and simple formulae shown in the box. Note that the contribution to the overall retention value from the different compartments has to be weighted by their individual blood flows. As can be understood the equation is under-determined, that is, there are more unknowns than knowns. A number of combinations of ventilation and perfusion values can fit the measured retention and excretion values. The single solution that is obtained by the mathematical analysis has, however, been shown to give a reliable description of the $\dot{V}_A/\dot{Q}$ distribution, both in theoretical experiments[10] and in animal and human studies, when the results have been compared with those from other techniques.[11][12] Using linear programming and Monte Carlo simulation, Evans and Wagner[13] presented a technique for defining the boundaries of a $\dot{V}_A/\dot{Q}$ distribution for a given set of retention and excretion data. Depending on the basic $\dot{V}_A/\dot{Q}$ pattern, the boundaries will be more or less narrow. Thus, a unimodal narrow $\dot{V}_A/\dot{Q}$ distribution has very tight boundaries, whereas a broad distribution of $\dot{V}_A/\dot{Q}$ ratios will be less precisely defined.

The inert gas mixture is prepared by bubbling three of the gases—SF_6, ethane, and cyclopropane—into an infusion bag of physiological saline. The bag is shaken vigorously for 1 minute and the excess gas removed. The procedure is carried out twice. The liquids—enflurane, ether, and acetone—are added thereafter and the saline bag is shaken again to mix all

---

Fig. 19.3   The principles of multiple inert gas elimination technique (MIGET). (a) Gas dissolved in blood will be partly eliminated via the airways when entering the pulmonary capillary. How much is retained in arterial blood is linearly related to the solubility (or the blood:gas partition coefficient, λ) and inversely related to the $\dot{V}_A/\dot{Q}$ ratio. Thus, gas with a high solubility in blood will be retained more than gas with a low solubility, and regions with a low $\dot{V}_A/\dot{Q}$ ratio will increase the retention of the gas, compared with regions with higher $\dot{V}_A/\dot{Q}$ ratios. (Shunt will cause all gas to be retained.) (b) Retention (R) and excretion (E) curves fitted to the measured values of six infused gases with different solubilities in blood. The broken curve has been fitted to the measured values according to the least squares method. The solid curve shows the retention and excretion in a hypothetical lung that is uniformly ventilated and perfused with a $\dot{V}_A/\dot{Q}$ ratio equal to the mean $\dot{V}_A/\dot{Q}$ of the lungs under study. The retention of the least soluble gas is near zero in a normal lung and the other gases are increasingly retained, in proportion to their λ value. Acetone is retained to almost 100%. The excretion ratios are lower than for the retention, an effect of the mixing with dead space gas. In the normal lung the measured and ideal R and E curves are close to each other. (c) The derived $\dot{V}_A/\dot{Q}$ distribution from the retention and excretion data shown in the left panel. A good match between ventilation ($\circ$) and perfusion ($\bullet$) can be seen, centred on a $\dot{V}_A/\dot{Q}$ ratio of $1\cdot0$.

the gases. The infusion is then started at a rate of 3–5 ml/min in adults, less in children and smaller experimental animals. After about 40 minutes of infusion, a steady state is reached and arterial and mixed venous blood samples are collected, together with a mixed expired gas sample, for subsequent analysis. As some of the gases are poorly soluble and others are

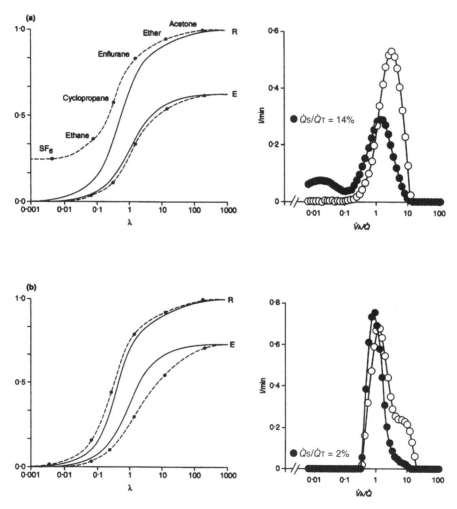

Fig 19.4   Examples of $\dot{V}_A/\dot{Q}$ mismatch: (a) increased retention of SF_6, an effect of the presence of shunt. There is also an increased retention of the moderately soluble gases (ethane, cyclopropane, enflurane) caused by the presence of low $\dot{V}_A/\dot{Q}$ regions. The most soluble gas (acetone) is hardly influenced by shunt and low $\dot{V}_A/\dot{Q}$ ratio and is retained to almost 100%. The excretion curve is less affected. (b) Decreased excretion of moderately soluble gases, caused by the presence of regions ventilated in excess of their perfusion ("high $\dot{V}_A/\dot{Q}$" regions). (o) Ventilation; (•) perfusion.

156

Basic equations for retentions of inert gases and the MIGET

The elimination of a gas ($\dot{V}$gas) from lung capillaries to exhaled air can be written according to equations (1) and (2).

$$\dot{V}\text{gas} = \dot{Q} + S(P\bar{v} - Pc') \tag{1}$$

where $\dot{Q}$ = pulmonary blood flow (cardiac output), S = solubility, $P\bar{v}$ = mixed venous gas tension, Pc' = end capillary gas tension.

$$\dot{V}\text{gas} = \frac{\dot{V}_A \times P_A}{Pb - P_{H_2O}} \tag{2}$$

where $\dot{V}_A$ = alveolar ventilation, P_A = alveolar gas tension, Pb = barometric pressure, P_{H_2O} = water vapour pressure ($P\bar{v}$, Pc', and P_A relate to the inert gas under study).

Combining eqns (1) and (2):

$$\frac{\dot{V}_A \times P_A}{Pb - P_{H_2O}} = \dot{Q} \times S(P\bar{v} - Pc') \tag{3}$$

$$\lambda = \frac{S}{Pb - P_{H_2O}}$$

where λ = blood:gas partition coefficient. Replacing S by λ:

$$\dot{V}_A \times P_A = \lambda \times \dot{Q}(P\bar{v} - Pc') \tag{4}$$

By rearranging:

$$R = \frac{P_A}{P\bar{v}} = \frac{\lambda}{\lambda + \dot{V}_A/\dot{Q}} \tag{5}$$

where R = retention.

For a multicompartmental analysis, the individual contributions will be perfusion weighted.

$$\frac{Pa}{P\bar{v}} = \sum_{j=1}^{j=n} \left[\frac{\lambda \times \dot{Q}j}{\lambda + (\dot{V}_A/\dot{Q})j} \right] \tag{6}$$

where j compartments are numbered from 1 to n.

Similarly, the excretion (E) can be calculated:

$$\frac{P_E}{P\bar{v}} = \sum_{j=1}^{j=n} \left[\frac{\lambda \times \dot{V}_Aj}{\lambda \times (\dot{V}_A/\dot{Q})j} \right] \tag{7}$$

where P_E = mixed expired gas tension. (Other symbols are explained above.)

soluble in fat and rubber, considerable precautions have to be taken when the samples are collected. Thus, glass syringes with matched barrels and plungers are the best choice for collection of the samples. The expired gas is passed through a heated metal mixing box.

For gas analysis, a gas chromatograph is normally used, although highly sensitive mass spectrometers have also been tested. These analyses require the blood sample to be measured using a tonometer, with a gas phase that can subsequently be entered into the analyser. This procedure consists of aspirating gas into two blood syringes, usually 8–10 ml N_2 to 6 ml blood. The syringes are then put in a heated shaking bath to ensure equilibration between the blood and gas phases. Through knowledge of the blood:gas partition coefficient and the gas and blood volumes (and the amount of anticoagulant), the initial amount in the blood sample can be calculated.

The gas chromatograph is equipped with a gas sampling loop with a switch, which transfers the gases into capillary columns that are 2 metres long, with a continuous gas flow, where the gases are separated. SF_6 is analysed by means of an electron capture detector and the other five gases by a flame ionisation detector. For this the column has to have the end divided into two branches, feeding each detector. As only the ratio between the blood and gas concentrations is needed, no calibration of the chromatograph is required, except for linearity tests.

Although the most reproducible results are obtained if a full set of samples is taken (arterial, mixed venous, and mixed expired) (Fig 19.5), the pulmonary arterial blood sample can be excluded if cardiac output, O_2 consumption ($\dot{V}O_2$), and CO_2 output ($\dot{V}CO_2$) are measured. This enables computation of the mixed venous gas concentrations by applying Fick's principle. Finally, the arterial sample can be substituted with peripheral venous blood. This requires a longer infusion time to achieve steady state— about 90 min—and the reproducibility may be lower than for a complete test.[14] The simplifications may, however, make the MIGET more attractive in clinical situations. For further information on the practical aspects of the method, see Wagner and Lopez.[14]

As a result of the assumptions and constraints that are needed for transforming the retention/excretion data to a multicompartment $\dot{V}A/\dot{Q}$ distribution, other approaches have been made to quantify the $\dot{V}A/\dot{Q}$ mismatch. Thus, methods have been described that are based on the calculation of the area between the measured and homogeneous retention and excretion curves.[15 16] These alternative approaches have, however, been used to a very limited extent.

Arterial–alveolar nitrogen difference

Another approach to calculate the perfusion of low $\dot{V}A/\dot{Q}$ regions is to measure the difference in arterial–alveolar N_2 tension. The method is based on the fact that, in lung units where the exchange rates of O_2 and CO_2 are not equal, the N_2 fraction in blood is altered from that of the inspired gas. In alveoli with a low $\dot{V}_A/\dot{Q}$ ratio, the N_2 tension rises almost in parallel with the decrease in P_{O_2} (the simultaneous change in P_{CO_2} can be no greater than the small difference in venous and arterial blood). This generates an arterial–alveolar N_2 difference. Moreover, this difference is not influenced by shunt blood, because that blood is not participating in any gas exchange. The technique has been tested in critically ill patients and compared with MIGET.[17] A fair correlation between the amount of low $\dot{V}_A/\dot{Q}$ ratio by MIGET and the arterial–alveolar N_2 difference was found as well as between shunt by MIGET and the difference between venous admixture (oxygen technique) and the arterial–alveolar N_2 difference. A limitation to the technique is the difficulty in measuring N_2 in blood, which is based on a manual gas absorption technique.

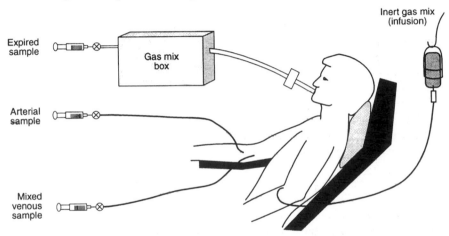

Fig 19.5 The technical set up for an inert gas study. The inert gases are dissolved in saline and infused at a slow rate to obtain the steady state condition. This normally takes about 40 min. Once steady state has been reached, however, a change in the conditions, for example, from rest to exercise, will result in a new steady state being reached within 10–15 min. For a full set of data, an arterial blood sample and a mixed venous blood sample (pulmonary artery) are collected simultaneously by drawing about 6 ml into heparinised, gas tight, glass syringes. Any gas bubble that might have been aspirated into the syringe should not be eliminated, but is used together with additional gas for the tonometering procedure. An expired gas sample is collected shortly after the blood samples to compensate for the delay in time through the gas mixing system. A simplified technique that does not require a mixed venous sample can also be used. In this case cardiac output has to be measured or assumed, to enable calculation of the mixed venous gas concentrations by the mass balance principle. Finally, the technique can be further simplified by replacing the arterial sample by a peripheral venous sample. This requires a longer infusion time to reach steady state, and a correction factor has to be introduced to compensate for gas losses in the periphery.[9]

Scintigraphic techniques

The ventilation and perfusion distributions can also be assessed by isotope techniques which give a spatial resolution. Ventilation may be assessed by breathing a radioactive gas or inhalation of radiolabelled aerosols or particles, as discussed in chapter 15.

The perfusion distribution is studied by embolisation, in the pulmonary vascular bed, of radiolabelled particles, either macroaggregated albumin (MAA) or microspheres of polystyrene, or other material.[18] The particle size is about 15–40 μm and an ordinary dose contains 200 000–500 000 particles. This should be compared with the almost 300×10^6 arterioles in which the particles are lodged. No measurable effect on vascular pressures should therefore be expected.

With positron emission tomography (PET), the local blood flow, ventilation, ventilation–perfusion ratios, permeability to proteins, density of receptors, and many other biologically relevant aspects may be estimated in vivo. Dynamic processes may be investigated with PET. The technique is based on principles developed for conventional x ray computed tomography and measures the distribution and biological behaviour of a variety of compounds labelled with positron emitting isotopes, such as ^{15}O, ^{11}C, ^{18}F, ^{13}N.[19] These positrons (positively charged anti-particles of electrons) typically have half lives of from a few seconds up to few minutes. An interaction with a tissue electron occurs usually within a distance of 1–5 mm, resulting in the emission of γ rays travelling at a 180° angle to each other. These γ rays are registered simultaneously by two detectors operating together.[19] A few investigations of $\dot{V}A/\dot{Q}$ with PET have been performed in awake humans.[20 21]

1 West JB. State of the art. Ventilation–perfusion relationships. *Am Rev Respir Dis* 1977;**116**:919–43.
2 Enghoff H. Volumen inefficax. Bemerkungen zur Frage des schädlichen Raumes. *Uppsala Läk För Förh* 1938;**44**:191.
3 Nunn JF. *Nunn's applied respiratory physiology*, 4th edn. Oxford: Heinemann 1993: 404–7.
4 Berggren S. The oxygen deficit of arterial blood caused by non-ventilating parts of the lung. *Acta Physiol Scand Suppl* 1942:1–92.
5 Murray JF, Davidson FF, Glazier JB. Modified technique for measuring pulmonary shunts using xenon and indocyanine green. *J Appl Physiol* 1972;**32**:695–700.
6 Jolin-Carlsson Å, Hedenstierna G, Blomqvist H, Strandberg Å. Separate lung blood flow in anesthetized dogs: A comparative study between electromagnetometry and SF_6 and CO_2 elimination. *Anesthesiology* 1987;**67**:240–6.
7 Wagner PD, Saltzman HA, West JB. Measurement of continuous distributions of ventilation–perfusion ratios: theory. *J Appl Physiol* 1974;**36**:588–99.
8 West JB, Wagner PD. Ventilation–perfusion relationships. In: Crystal RG, West JB, eds. *The lung, scientific foundations*, 2nd edn. New York: Lippincott Raven, 1997: 1693–709.
9 Wagner PD, Smith CM, Davies NJH, McEvoy RD, Gale GE. Estimation of ventilation–perfusion inequality by inert gas elimination without arterial sampling. *J Appl Physiol* 1985;**59**:376–83.
10 Wagner PD. Calculation of the distribution of ventilation–perfusion ratios from inert gas elimination data. *Fed Proc* 1982;**41**:136–9.

11 Hedenstierna G, White FC, Mazzone R, Wagner PD. Redistribution of pulmonary blood flow in the dog with PEEP ventilation. *J Appl Physiol* 1979;**46**:278–87.
12 Tokics L, Hedenstierna G, Svensson L, Brismar B, Cederlund T, Lundquist H, Strandberg Å. V/Q distribution and correlation to atelectasis in anesthetized paralyzed humans. *J Appl Physiol* 1996;**81**:1822–33.
13 Evans JW, Wagner PD. Limits on VA/Q distributions from analysis of experimental inert gas elimination. *J Appl Physiol* 1977;**42**:889–98.
14 Wagner PD, Lopez FA. Gas chromatography techniques in respiratory physiology. *Respir Physiol* 1984;**403**:1–24.
15 Hlastala MP, Robertson HT. Inert gas elimination characteristics of the normal and abnormal lung. *J Appl Physiol* 1978;**44**:258–66.
16 Neufeld GR, Williams JJ, Klineberg PL, Marshall BE. Inert gas a–v differences: a direct reflection of V/Q distribution. *J Appl Physiol* 1978;**44**:277–83.
17 Radermacher P, Hérigault R, Teisseire B, Harf A, Lemaire F. Low V_A/Q areas: arterial–alveolar N_2 difference and multiple inert gas elimination technique. *J Appl Physiol* 1988;**64**:2224–9.
18 Tow DE, Wagner HN Jr, Lopez-Majano V, Smith EM, Migita T. Validity of measuring regional pulmonary arterial blood flow with macroaggregates of human serum albumin. *Am J Roentgenol Radium Ther Nucl Med* 1966;**96**:664–76.
19 Hughes JMB, Coates G. Radionuclide imaging: positron camera. In: Potchen EJ, Grainger R, Green R, eds. *Pulmonary radiology*. Philadelphia: WB Saunders, 1993: 331–9.
20 Brudin LH, Rhodes CG, Valind SO, Jones T, Hughes JMB. Interrelationships between regional blood flow, blood volume and ventilation in supine man. *J Appl Physiol* 1994;**76**:1205–10.
21 Rhodes CG, Valind SO, Brudin LH, Wollmer PE, Jones T, Buckingham PD, Hughes JMB. Quantification of regional V_A/Q ratios in humans by use of PET. II. Procedure and normal values. *J Appl Physiol* 1989;**66**:1905–13.

20: Reference values

The measurement of lung function requires that the observed value can be related to something that has been defined as normal or, alternatively, pathological. There are large reference materials with normal values for most lung function variables. Mostly, there is not a single value that can be considered the normal reference, but sex, age, height, and weight affect what should be considered normal in a particular subject. Therefore multiple regression equations have been constructed for the determination of the reference value. More fancy equations have also been constructed to fit a function to measured data. When logarithmic, exponential, quadratic, hyperbolic, and other functions are applied, it should be possible to explain, on biological or physiological grounds, why such a function has been adapted to measured data

The predicted reference value is usually the arithmetic mean of several observations, or the value given by a regression function, fitted to the observed data. There is a certain range of observations of equally "normal" data around the mean, or along the regression line. It is generally considered that values that are within two standard deviations (SD) of the mean should be judged as normal. By this means, 95% of all observations in a study group that has been considered healthy with respect to the studied variable have a "normal" value. More interesting might be the fact that 5% of this "normal" population will have abnormal values. Moreover, a patient with lung disease may present with a value within normal limits. He or she may have had a lung function value that was two SD above the reference before the disease, and it may fall by as much as four SD before it is outside the range of "normal". Obviously, it is easier to detect an abnormality by following the patient with repeated lung function measurements, than by making one measurement and comparing the result with a reference value.

When following a patient over a long time period, it must be remembered that the reference value may also change, because it is affected by age and body dimensions. Thus, a decrease in a variable may solely reflect the normal ageing process and not any disease.

Finally, body position may affect the lung function and, hence, what should be considered normal. For example, functional residual capacity (FRC) is reduced in the supine position, compared with standing. Most reference values have been obtained in the upright position which must be remembered when interpreting results that may have been obtained in another body position.

To obtain the reference value, the sex, age, and often also the height and weight have to be entered into a computer program or a table. A number of frequently used regression equations for reference values of different lung function variables can be found in the further reading cited below.

Further reading

General: variables, methods, units

Cotes JE, Chinn DJ, Quanjer PH, Roca J, Yernault JC. Standardization of the measurement of transfer factor (diffusing capacity). Report of Working Party "Standardization of Lung Function Tests", European Community for Steel and Coal. Official Statement of the European Respiratory Society [see comments]. *Eur Respir J Suppl* 1993;**16**:41–52.

Quanjer PH, Dalhuijsen A, van Zomeren BC. Reference populations: general data. Regression equations for reference values. In: Quanjer PH, ed. Standardized lung function testing. Report of Working Party "Standardization of Lung Function Tests". *Bull Eur Physiopathol Respir* 1983;**19**(suppl 5):1–95.

Quanjer PH, Tammeling GJ, Cotes JE, Fabbri LM, Matthys H, Pedersen OF, et al. Symbols, abbreviations and units. Working Party "Standardization of Lung Function Tests", European Community for Steel and Coal. *Eur Respir J Suppl* 1993;**16**:85–100.

Reference values for lung volumes and forced spirometry

Crapo RO, Morris AH. Standardized single breath normal values for carbon monoxide diffusing capacity. *Am Rev Respir Dis* 1981;**123**:185–9.

Crapo RO, Morris AH, Gardner RM. Reference spirometric values using techniques and equipment that meet ATS recommendations. *Am Rev Respir Dis* 1981;**123**:659–64.

Hedenström H, Malmberg P, Agarwal K. Reference values for lung function tests in females. Regression equations with smoking variables. *Bull Eur Physiopathol Respir* 1985;**21**:551–7.

Hedenström H, Malmberg P, Fridriksson HV. Reference values for lung function tests in men: regression equations with smoking variables. *Upps J Med Sci.* 1986;**91**:299–310.

Knudson RJ, Lebowitz MD, Holberg CJ, Burrows B. Changes in the normal maximal expiratory flow-volume curve with growth and aging. *Am Rev Respir Dis* 1983;**127**:725–34.

Stocks J, Quanjer PH. Reference values for residual volume, functional residual capacity and total lung capacity. ATS Workshop on Lung Volume Measurements. Official Statement of The European Respiratory Society. *Eur Respir J* 1995;**8**:492–506.

Reference values for gas distribution indices and airway closure

Becklake MR. A new index of the intrapulmonary mixture of inspired air. *Thorax.* 1952;7:111–16.

Buist AS, Ross BB. Predicted values for closing volumes using a modified single breath nitrogen test. *Am Rev Respir Dis* 1973;**107**:744–52.

Buist AS, Ross BB. Quantitative analyses of the alveolar plateau in the diagnosis of early airway obstruction. *Am Rev Respir Dis* 1973; **108**:1078–87.

Cumming G, Guyatt GR. Alveolar gas mixing efficiency in the human lung. *Clini Sci* 1982;**62**:541–7.

Fowler WS, Cornish ER Jr, Kety S. Lung function studies. VIII. Analysis of alveolar ventilation by pulmonary N_2 clearance curves. *J Clin Invest* 1952;31:40–50.

Reference values for respiratory mechanics

Hedenström H, Malmberg P, Agarwal K. Reference values for lung function tests in females. Regression equations with smoking variables. *Bull Eur Physiopathol Respir* 1985;**21**:551–7.

Hedenström H, Malmberg P, Fridriksson HV. Reference values for lung function tests in men: regression equations with smoking variables. *Upps J Med Sci* 1986;**91**:299–310.

Noseda A, Van Muylem A, Estenne M, Yernault JC. Inspiratory and expiratory lung pressure-volume curve in healthy males and females. *Bull Eur Physiopathol Respir* 1984;**20**:245–9

Paiva M, Yernault JC, Van Eedeweghe P, Englert M. A sigmoid model of the static volume–pressure curve of human lung. *Respir Physiol* 1975; **23**:317–23.

Reference values for children

Paoletti P, Viegi G, Pistelli G, Di Pede F, Fazzi P, Polato R, et al. Reference equations for the single-breath diffusing capacity. *Am Rev Respir Dis* 1985;**132**:806–13.

Quanjer PH, Helms P, Bjure J, Gaultier C. Standardization of lung function tests in paediatrics. *Eur Respir J Suppl* 1989;**2**(suppl 4):1–264.

Quanjer PH, Stocks J, Polgar G, Wise M, Karlberg J, Borsboom G. Compilation of reference values for lung function measurements in children. *Eur Respir J Suppl* 1989;**2**(suppl 4):184–261.

Solymar L, Aronsson P, Bake B, Bjure J. Nitrogen single-breath test, flow–volume curves and spirometry in healthy children 7–18 years of age. *Eur J Respir Dis* 1980;**61**:275–86.

Glossary

$\text{A}-\text{a}P\text{O}_2$	alveolar–arterial $P\text{O}_2$ difference
$C\text{a}$	arterial blood gas concentration
$C\bar{\text{v}}$	mixed venous gas concentration
CC	closing capacity
$C\text{cw}$	chest wall compliance
$C\text{lung}$	lung compliance
$C\text{rs}$	total respiratory compliance
COPD	chronic obstructive pulmonary disease
CV	closing volume
$D\text{LCO}$	CO diffusing capacity
$D\text{LO}_2$	oxygen diffusing capacity
FEF_{50}, FEF_{75}	forced espiratory flow at 50% and 75% respectively of expired FVC (used in the USA)
$\text{FEV}_\%$	FEV_1/VC
FEV_1	forced expiratory volume in 1 second
$F\text{IO}_2$	fractional concentration of inspired oxygen
$\text{FIV}_\%$	FIV_1/FIVC
FIV_1	forced inspiratory volume in 1 second
FIVC	forced inspired vital capacity
FRC	functional residual capacity
FVC	forced vital capacity
MEF	maximum expiratory flow
MEF_{25}, etc	maximum expiratory flow with 25% of VC remaining
MEF_{50}, MEF_{25}	maximum midexpiratory flow or forced expiratory flow with 50% and 25% of FVC remaining (symbols used in Europe, corresponding to FEF_{50} and FEF_{75} in the USA)
$P\text{aO}_2$, $P\text{aCO}_2$	arterial gas tension
$P\text{AO}_2$, $P\text{ACO}_2$	alveolar gas tension
$Pc'\text{O}_2$, $Pc'\text{CO}_2$	end capillary gas tension
$P\text{Emax}$	maximum expiratory (alveolar) pressure
$P\bar{\text{E}}\text{O}_2$, $P\bar{\text{E}}\text{CO}_2$	mixed expired gas tension
$P\text{ETO}_2$, $P\text{ETCO}_2$	end tidal gas tension
$P\text{Imax}$	maximum inspiratory (alveolar) pressure
$P\text{IO}_2$	inspired oxygen tension

$P\bar{v}_{O_2}$, $P\bar{v}_{CO_2}$	mixed venous gas tension
Paw	airway pressure
Palv	alveolar gas pressure
P_B	barometric pressure
PEEP	positive end expiratory pressure
$PEEP_i$	intrinsic PEEP
PEF	peak expiratory flow
Poes	oesophageal pressure
Ppl	pleural pressure
Pst	elastic recoil pressure
Ptp	transpulmonary pressure
Pw	chest wall recoil pressure
$\dot{Q}$c	capillary flow
$\dot{Q}$s	shunt
$\dot{Q}$s/$\dot{Q}_T$	shunt fraction
$\dot{Q}_T$	cardiac output
Raw	airway resistance
Rlung tis	lung tissue resistance
Rtot	total respiratory resistance
RV	residual volume
Rw	chest wall resistance
T_{LCO}	CO transfer factor
TLC	total lung capacity
$\dot{V}$	ventilation
V_A	alveolar volume
$\dot{V}_A$	alveolar ventilation
$\dot{V}_A/\dot{Q}$	ventilation-perfusion ratio
VC	vital capacity
V_D	volume of dead space
V_D/V_T	proportion of tidal volume ventilating dead space
V_T	tidal volume
$\dot{V}_{CO_2}$	carbon dioxide output
$\dot{V}_{O_2}$	oxygen consumption

166

Index